Acid Reflux Diet
And Cookbook

The new complete guide to prevent gastric acid, a
healthy diet with quick and easy recipes

Charles Thompson

Copyright © 2020 by Charles Thompson

Contents

Introduction

Acid reflux is a common digestive condition that creates irritation, heartburn, and pain at the opening of the stomach as well as burning in the food canal. A person experiences this issue due to the reverse flow of the fluid and food from the stomach towards the throat. All over the world, people commonly face acid reflux and other related issues, which can be worse if not treated on time and properly. According to health consultants, the increased ratio of acid reflux issues is due to inappropriate food consumption, poor food options, lack of sleep, stressful mental conditions, and lack of physical activity in people's everyday routine. The digestive system is a sensitive part of the body and can be easily disturbed due to any physical exertion or mental restlessness.

The continuous problem with gastric issues can influence a person's productivity and thinking ability. It can restrict a person's activities and can be the cause of severe ulcer or esophageal cancer as well. the best and most natural way to treat acid reflux and its complications is a change of lifestyle. Following proper diet plans and implementing exercise routines can help a person to overcome the reflux and improve their digestive health. People with obesity, diabetes, or who have inflammation issues can easily be affected by acid reflux. According to doctors, it is recommended that to overcome and avoid the gastric acid reflux, a person should maintain a healthy weight and keep active for at least 30 to 40 minutes at a time on a regular basis.

This book provides enough information about acid reflux, its causes, symptoms and treatment options. As well as for the reader, it has the information that reveals how lifestyle changes can improve a person's overall health and reduce the signs and complications of acid reflux. For those with diet concerns, we have included some healthy and delicious recipes for those who are living with acid reflux. This way, those struggling with this issue can still have or enjoy the delicious food. It has many other interesting and informative facts about acid reflux and how to treat this condition with natural, healthy food.

Chapter 1:
Gastric Acid Reflux

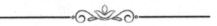

The human body is a complex one that is crafted very well. Everything is connected to each other and all the organs or tissues are working in perfect synchronization. If one thing goes wrong, then it will put a direct effect on the rest of the body as well. Our stomach is one of the integral organs of the body that affects many other parts as well. If your stomach is not working as it should, then your skin will be dull, and you will have acne, scars, heartburn, bloating, pain and a feeling of unrest. Among all these things, you may feel acid reflux in the body.

Acid reflux is a condition of having a burning pain that is similar to heartburn in lower chest or sometimes your food pipe or throat as well. When the stomach acid flows upward to the food pipe, it causes the acidic feeling to the pipe and lower chest. Sometimes in severe conditions is can come up to the throat, cause severe pain, and make you uncomfortable.

It seems to be a commonly experienced feeling by a majority of people in their daily routine, sometimes once in a week and sometimes in every 15 to 20 days. A person is diagnosed with the gastric acid reflux when he or she is experiencing the feeling more than twice a week. In such conditions, it is necessary for the person to move forward and ask for medical help.

Causes

Before heading for a doctor, it is necessary to look into the causes of acid reflux. Whenever our body is not functioning properly or an organ is behaving differently, there are certain reasons behind that. It is important to identify these reasons and problems in the first place. When you know the causes, you will be able to move toward a better treatment and prevention system. Therefore, here we are, discussing some of the major causes that lead to acid reflux.

Hiatus or Hernia

One of the non-preventable causes of acid reflux is the Hiatus or Hernia. It is a condition when a hole occurs in diaphragm that leads to the upper part of the stomach to enter the chest cavity. This situation can cause the acid from stomach to reflux in the upper canal and cause the burning sensation in throat and chest section.

It is one of the critical conditions in overall human health, as the person will not be able to control the factor. Only a surgery and proper treatment to the hernia can help to avoid the gastric acid reflux in such conditions. There is a 100 percent chance of acid reflux in hernia patients, as both sections intersect one other in this situation.

Obesity

Another cause of gastric acid reflux is obesity. When there is a lack of weight management, then our body behaves differently. Weight that is above average has an intense reaction in the body. Organs start behaving differently and this can result in issues. Obesity is not a normal condition; in fact, it is connected to a number of health risks. Increased weight and body mass affect total body stamina, bone strength, heart performance, blood circulation, hormonal changes and organ activities.

Gastric acid reflux is one of the major outcomes that are related to obesity. The stomach is unable to digest all the food properly, and the acid release is an effort to deal with the excessive energy left in the body. It causes the outward flow of acid from the stomach. Moreover, obesity can affect the stomach size and its movement can trigger the condition of acid reflux.

Smoking

Smoking is one of the biggest causes of acid reflux. It is a known fact that cigarettes and cigars have acidic reactions in the body. Moreover, smoking affects the overall organ system composition as well. It can not only affect the lungs, but the stomach as well. In response to the smoke and all the chemicals in it, the acid in the stomach reaches the food canal in reverse. When the person inhales and exhales smoke, it can come up with fumes of acid from the stomach and can increase the risks and effects of gastric acid reflux.

Alcohol

Another major cause of acid reflux is the use of alcohol. Alcoholism is dangerous for a person's overall health. It affects the lifestyle and internal organs of the body. The consumption of alcohol is good if kept within a safe limit, but when there is excessive use, there will be problems. Acid reflux is one of the problems that are caused as a result of excessive alcohol consumption.

The important thing is to keep the consumption of alcohol in normal routine and keep it limited for the safe use.

No or low physical activity

The food we eat is digested in our stomach and the process is triggered by two major things. One is acid, and the other is physical activity. If a person eats and has no or low physical activity, then there can be a chance of acid reflux. The stomach will produce acid in order to digest food, but the excessive amount of acid will produce a reflux in the food canal in the event of no activity. It is important to have a walk after a meal or exert your body physically to trigger the proper digestion of your food. It will help you to make things better and smooth as well. Physical activity will help you to make the better use of acid in the stomach and get it dissolved in the food. It will neutralize the acid in the digestion process and will get you all the necessary nutrients you need.

Multiple drugs and sedatives

Sometimes the sedative medications and anti-depressant drugs we take can cause acidity in the stomach. That acidity can lead to ultimate gastric acid reflux. It is necessary to have a safe and limited dosage of the drugs. The excessive use of medicine, especially without prescriptions, could affect your overall stomach functions.

Pregnancy

During pregnancy, there are numerous changes that occur. From mood swings to food options and psychological ideas to physical movements, everything changes. During this process, females have threats to face, many of them being critical health constraints. It can happen sometimes due to lack of care, vitamins, or excessive use of a specific product. There are sometimes the genetic reactions in the body as well. Acid reflux is something that is not inherited, but it can be caused by pregnancy and body changes. Your stomach may behave differently and you may not be getting as physical movement, so it can lead to a reflux situation.

Moreover, the vomiting and constant nausea caused by pregnancy can always trigger the gastric acid reflux. In this regard, the important thing is to monitor everything and then have essential solutions.

Poor dietary selection

Your food intake and dietary choices matter a lot when it comes to your overall health. Acid reflux can be triggered by poor dietary options. If you are consuming junk food, soft drinks, dried snacks, and fat rich food options then you may feel the hits of acid reflux. Such food options increase the acidity in the stomach and can result in issues.

Improper posture after meal

Acid reflux is not just caused by medical deficiencies and complications. In fact, it can come up as a reaction to bad posture . It is necessary to ensure the proper physical posture when having meal. Bending over your waist or lying on your back while eating or right after taking meal can result in acid reflux. It can be dangerous and build up the issue for more serious causes. It is necessary to watch out during your meal and pay attention to your movement routine in order to avoid such drastic outcomes from your activities.

Bedtime snacks

Bedtime snacking is one of the common habits that people have. It is a kind of regular routine for people in many cases. On the other hand, it is one of the critical causes of acid reflux. Eating food at bedtime does not allow it to digest properly, and the physical posture that often accompanies bedtime snacking can cause the stomach acids to reflux upwards.

Symptoms

Most people confuse gastric acid reflux with heartburn. Sometimes it is claimed that both are same and sometimes they are marked as different. Although there is a fine line difference between the two, it is necessary to underline the difference focusing on the symptoms of acid reflux. You can fight with a medical condition after knowing its causes and major symptoms. The symptoms are necessary for the better evaluation and diagnosis.

Acid reflux is one of the conditions that people do not take seriously in the beginning. Lately, when things are a bit out of control, they became concerned about the issue. In order to live healthily, the important thing is to keep the symptoms and all changes in the body under consideration. It is good to know the major symptoms and take note of these symptoms. Eventually, it will help in self and early diagnosis and then you can come up with the best of remedies and treatments. Here are a few major symptoms of gastric acid reflux to consider:

- ❖ Heartburn is one of the major symptoms of acid reflux. It is not the same thing, but the first step that leads to the condition. You can feel a discomfort or pain with a burning sensation in your abdomen and chest area that goes up to your throat.
- ❖ Bitter tasting in back side of mouth and throat is another symptom that is shows the bad stomach condition and acid reflux
- ❖ Burning sensation in the upper throat can be a reaction of acid reflux
- ❖ You can feel nausea and an ultimate feeling of throwing up the food you just had
- ❖ Continuous burping with a bad smell and acidic feeling
- ❖ Vomit can be bloody and painful in severe cases
- ❖ Acid reflux can cause black and bloody stools, accompanied by a burning sensation

- There can be difficult hiccups with a mixed feeling of pain and burning
- The immense reduction in weight can be observed without any reason
- Sore throat, dry cough, and wheezing can occur in initial and chronic stages of acid reflux
- There can be a feeling of unease in the throat, like food is stuck in the throat and will be out in no time
- Difficulty in swallowing food, with pain and burning
- Bad breath and dental erosion are other major symptoms of acid reflux

The condition of acid reflux not only affects the stomach and causes a burning sensation inside. In fact, it leads to some major outcomes. If there is not proper treatment of the condition, then results can be drastic. It can start as a simple problem of indigestion or acidity in the stomach that will lead to burping and even up resulting in bloody vomit, difficulty in swallowing and much more. It is necessary to identify these basic symptoms initially and take measures in order to resolve these issues quickly.

You can get to know more symptoms of acid reflux in certain cases. It is not necessary that everyone will face the same issues in the beginning. The person could have any of these or all of these symptoms from time to time. The best way is to be alert with the treatment, even if you are facing the initial or minor symptoms. Sometimes you may have these issues mixed with any other health condition, then make sure to discuss this with your physician in the first place.

Remember, bad smell and throat issues largely come from your stomach, and if these go unnoticed, then you may have to face the music. Note the symptoms and related symbols of the problem and consider these things in your daily routine for early diagnosis and control of the problem.

Treatments

Gastric acid reflux seems to be a common and normal issue. However, in extreme cases,, it can be lethal. If you are ignoring the condition and not concerned about getting treatment, you will still have to face the issues in the end. Whenever a person is suffering from the acid reflux, it is necessary to go for the treatment and remedies in the first place. Without a proper and organized treatment, it is not possible to recover from the condition, and it can cause issues in the long run. Here are some treatment options that one could consider.

Medications

During the initial stage when a person is facing issues with heartburn or acidity, there are certain medications to use to control these symptoms. It is necessary to use these medications after the proper consultation. Remember you may mix up heartburn and acid reflux with each other. Heartburn can be a condition in acid reflux, but it is not the acid reflux all the time.

Gaviscon is one of the famous and commonly used drugs to treat problems related to heartburn. It is one of the mild and effective sources that help to reduce the burning in the initial scale. If you have the severe case of acid reflux, then you will get the drugs in combination of famotidine, ranitidine, cimetidine, rebeprazole, omeprazole and others. Make sure to consult a physician in severe cases for the medication prescription and keep up with regular checkups.

Surgery

When it is not possible to treat the condition of acid reflux using medications, then doctors have another option: surgery. To treat conditions, there are two types of surgeries depending on the condition and the patient's situation. In the first type of surgical procedure, there is a placement of a LINX device around and outside the lowered end of the esophagus or food pipe. The device is made of titanium wires that work as a barrier to fluid flowing outward from the stomach. The device helps patients to quit or reduce medication intake. Having the device after a surgery comes with a number of limitations. For example, the patient can never have MRI test later on. Moreover, it is necessary to check if the patient is allergic to any metal or not.

The second surgical procedure is the fundoplication that helps to reduce the acid reflux. In the procedure, an artificial valve is attached to the top of stomach that wraps the upper part of the stomach and reduces the chances of acid reflux. It can be a treatment for the hiatal hernia as well.

Both of these surgical procedures should be considered a last resort in the case of acid reflux. The first preference in every case is prevention using lifestyle changes, the second is medication with major lifestyle changes. In the end, if the condition is critical and patient needs ultimate help, then surgery is the option that doctors should eventually resort to.

Lifestyle

Along with the medication or surgery when you are suffering from acid reflux, then you need to make some essential lifestyle changes. Adopting some of the right habits and making a difference in your routine will help you to be good and better with the treatment. Here are the major changes you need to make in your daily routine:

- ❖ Take a light and spice free diet
- ❖ Eat healthy and fresh
- ❖ Eat in intervals
- ❖ Take your medications on time
- ❖ Do not wear tight clothes or belts
- ❖ Take your meals in intervals and in small portions
- ❖ Increase your physical activity to help your body consume energy and reduce weight if you are overweight

Risks and Complications

If there is a lack of concern towards the issue and you delay treatment, then it can lead to some drastic complications. They can seem to be minor issues, but can never be so reckless that you must face the critical music. Here are the complications you may have to face:

- ❖ The borderline of the esophagus can be damaged and inflamed, causing constant irritation, internal bleeding, and ulceration in some cases.

- ❖ There can be a non-stop burning and internal irritation that can affect the overall health and enhance psychological pressure as well.

- ❖ There can be scar development that will lead to difficult swallowing and food will not be able to travel down the esophagus

- ❖ The repeated exposure of the cells and tissues to the stomach acid can change their formation. It can damage the cell structure, causing them to be dead and potentially leading to cancer development.

It is necessary to focus on the problem in the first stage in order to help with the proper treatment. In case of permanent negligence, things can be difficult to control and will come up with some of the ultimately damaging results as a whole.

Chapter 2:
Prevention of Acid Reflux

Prevention is better than treatment, as we all know. It is not just a phrase but in all matters, it is the ultimate solution and escape. No matter from what disease you are going through, you need to make sure that you will adopt some of the important preventions that will help you to live a healthy life.

In case of acid reflux, things are quite manageable and in your hand. There are certain preventions that help to keep your body in order. It is not something that is caused by any external virus or infection; it is all about the mismanagement in your daily routine. With a little management and care, you can stop or revert things in the initial stage. It is quite easy to follow the prevention guide for acid reflux.

What are some common preventions?

The preventions for acid reflux are more related to your food options than hygienic conditions. It is a kind of lifestyle problem that can occur and trigger to your mismanagement with food, posture, habits, and lifestyle as well. Therefore, it is necessary that you follow some safe lifestyle options in order to avoid further damage to your body.

Using the prevention options, you will be able to avoid the factors that can cause acid reflux, such as heartburn, obesity, depression, drugs, hernia and much more. In our body, everything is linked with each other and you have to make sure that your overall body is healthy. Overall health is something that can help you to be good in life and avoid all the serious threats and issues.

How Does Food Help?

All problems related to stomach are directly connected to food. The food or diet we use is one of the integral factors in our body. All the minerals and nutrients we get from our food helps us to grow. In case if we do not eat properly or have the right food that we need, it means we can have some deficiencies in the body as well. From the beginning of our lives, cycle doctors recommend having the best food and diet plan in general. There should be everything healthy and well-composed in terms of nutrition, so the body will not have any deficiencies at all.

We once took care of everything in the diet since the birth of a child. Other supplements for nutrition are for emergency use when only diet is not helping the situation. Therefore, in order to prevent acid reflux, we need to get help from food in the first place. It is one of the best resources that will help you throughout life to manage the symptoms of acid reflux. If you want to avoid acid reflux, food helps. If you want to treat acid reflux during the initial stage, food helps. If you have undergone surgery and are trying to maintain your condition, food helps. In short, no matter what your condition is, food is the factor that actually helps you to keep things in control. The question is how it can help you and what you can get out of it.

In order to prevent acid reflux using food therapy, it is necessary to make a food selection that helps you in the following manner:

Reduce acidity

It is necessary to eat food that reduces acidity and that does not have an acidic nature. As such, you cannot take coffee, alcohol, citrus and other foods that increase the acidic ratio in stomach. By taking the food that reduces acidity and that is lighter in nature, this will help your stomach to be better and reduce its acidic fluency. Moreover, it will not let the acid to reflux in the food pipe or cause burning in the stomach.

Provide the best nutrients

When you are recovering from acid reflux, your stomach is weak and it affects your overall body as well. You need to choose the food options with the best nutrients. Make sure to eat healthy food enriched with calcium, magnesium and phosphorus. Fruits like bananas, apples and berries help to reduce acidity. Make sure to avoid the processed food with many spices that can kill the nutrients in the food.

Reduce inflammation

Inflammation or burning is primarily caused by the unlimited spices and sauces we use in our food. It is necessary to take mild spices and sauces in order to keep your dietary choices light. The food spices can increase the burning sensation and double up the inflammation as well. You need to pick up food options with minimum spices or no spices in certain conditions. Moreover, choose to have anti-inflammatory food options that will help you to reduce the overall inflammation in the organs and body.

Helps to repair organs

There are food options like meat, white meat, grains, and sprouts that are enriched with protein and have the nature to repair body cells internally. The continuous acid reflux in the body causes the organs and cells to become damaged at a large scale. You need some extra nutrients to ensure the proper recovery of these cells and to have better health overall. In this manner, you need to pick up the food options that help in cell repairing and that makes you feel better from the inside out. It will be an overall benefit for you.

Keep the digestion process lighter

Some major issues with the acid reflux are with digestion. The acid in the stomach is produced to digest food when we eat so much acidic food that the acid's ratio gets higher and causes a reflux. In order to avoid such conditions, it is necessary to eat food that is lighter to digest. It will help the stomach to produce a lesser amount of acid and digest the food easily. Moreover, the food will not be acidic in nature so it will get mixed in the stomach acid and neutralize the overall equation. It is a little science but overall helps to avoid any critical condition that will make you suffer in future on a larger scale.

The best food options to reduce and prevent acid reflux

Not all healthy diet plans or food options are effective enough to help you with the acid reflux prevention and treatment. You need to pick up the specific combinations and safe food options that help to reduce inflammation, burning and acidity. Moreover, you need to keep a balance between your food intake so things will be balanced and work appropriately. Here are some major food options that you can use to prevent acid reflux or to have a quick recovery from the problem:

- ❖ Fresh vegetables that are rich in nutrients and low in fat and sugar
- ❖ Ginger
- ❖ Non-citrus fruits like banana, guava, apple, kiwi and more
- ❖ Lean meat and sea food
- ❖ Healthy fats like coconut oil, organic butter and more
- ❖ Egg whites

All these foods are not acidic in nature and reduce fats from the body. It is a good option to treat these foods as a priority. They can help in prevention and quick recovery from the acid reflux at the beginning. On the other hand, it's important to take a healthy diet seriously so that you can help your body to increase immunity and fight back these issues and problems.

Lifestyle Changes

In order to prevent acid reflux and have a quick recovery, in addition to controlling your diet, you need to make some lifestyle changes. These changes help bring about quick and effective recovery as well as prevention from the problem. These changes not only help to avoid the acid reflux problem but to have a better life and avoid any further health constraints.

Eat healthy

In your lifestyle changes, the very first thing you need to do is to eat healthy food. Even if you are eating processed meals, refined sugar, and other things, then make sure to substitute them with healthier alternatives. There should be an irregular pattern of the consumption of these food options. You need to make healthy food options your priority in order to avoid such issues and complications.

Plan your meals

Make sure to take your meals on time at specific intervals. Eating too much or having meals with long breaks in between can never be healthy. You need to feed your stomach with a small meal after a specific interval so there will be no acidity in there. The planned interval based meals will help you in the path toward safe digestion.

Get 8 hours of sleep

Sleep is important to let your food digest and your stomach to work efficiently. Make sure that you are taking healthy and good sleep for 8 hours each night. It should be a quality night of sleep for a continuous 8 hours, not in breaks or parts. In the case of a partial sleep cycle, you will feel more exhausted and drained in the end.

Manage your stress

Stress and anxiety can actually affect the digestion system of your stomach. It is not ideal for a healthy living if you keep stressing out your body. Make sure that you keep a balance between work life and leisure time in order to relax yourself and avoid any health complications. A stressful brain affects the overall body functions and can cause acid reflux.

Maintain a balance between food options

Lifestyle changes are not about quitting the food options and limiting yourself to a specific kind of diet. It is about balancing your food options. You need to keep the balance between the food options you want to have and that you can have. Make sure that you pick up the right options that will help you to maintain a good balance in your overall intake.

Do not sleep immediately after meals

It is not an ideal habit to sleep or lay down immediately after having a meal. In such conditions, it is not possible for the stomach to digest the food properly. It increases the chances of acid reflux and acidity in stomach to a maximum level.

Increase physical exertion

Laziness and being in one place for extended periods of time is one of the triggers for acid reflux. If you are not having good physical activity in your daily routine, that means you are not letting your energy get consumed. In such a situation, the stomach acid stays in the stomach and is not be able to dissolve properly. This can cause refluxes later on. With the help of physical exertion, you will be able to reduce your weight and the chances of acid reflux.

Impact of Exercise

In the prevention and basic treatment, along with food, lifestyle changes and exercise will have a great impact on your overall results. Exercise and good physical activity can help your body to avoid many complications. Exercise activates all your organs, muscles and tissues. It allows you to consume all the energy taken from the food. Moreover, the stomach will digest the food instantly and the acid will not stay in your stomach later on.

Lean muscles

By reducing the amount of fats you intake, you have more chances of living a healthy life. In order to be happy and stress free from any issues such as acid reflux, you need to have a healthy body. Regular exercise helps you to have the lean muscles that mean you will have less fats and other related problems. It will also reduce the chances of acidity in your body and allow you to consume all the energy from the food you consume food. Eventually, you can avoid many of the issues and problems related to acid reflux and other related problems.

Better organ functioning

When our body is in a resting position, it is not possible for all the organs to work efficiently. In the rest position or daily normal routine, not all your organs get the pressure and involved in the physical exertion. It causes these organs to have fats and face issues that can lead to some complications like acid reflux. Our stomach causes acid reflux because our stomach does not get the real word to do because of our inactivity. With the help of continuous efforts and activity, things can be better and you can avoid such problems.

Weight reduction

Obesity is one of the causes that triggers acid reflux. Workout and exercise not only helps keep your body healthy, but helps to reduce weight as well. It melts down all the fat from the body and gives you all good muscles and only muscular weight. On the other hand, it will help you to get better in the overall health scale so that you can enjoy your life.

Reduced inflammation

Exercise helps to break and make muscles and cells as well. The exertion activates the repairing muscles in the body that helps to reduce the internal and external inflammation. The acid reflux causes worse inflammation internally and makes the person unrestful. Exercise helps to deal with this painful condition and triggers the body to repair cells and damaged organs.

Active mind and healthy body

Along with food management, a good exercise routine is a perfect combination for a healthy body and active mind. By working out, you will consume all the excessive energy from the your food. Moreover it will release the stress and tension you have. In the end, you can have an active and peaceful mind with a lighter body. With all the exertion, our brain releases the stress hormones and eliminates them from the body in many ways.

Chapter 3:
Treatment & Complications

Gastric acid reflux is not a chronic disease and people usually feel reflux after having a certain food. It is normal in several cases and can be eliminated and reduced with certain medical or natural remedies. But if it is not treated well or a person is having some digestive system problem, the problem can be persistent and become worse. The chronic disease of acid reflux refers to gastroesophageal reflux diseases. It usually occurs when a person constantly feels acid or food between the canal tube that is linked between the stomach and throat. It is also known as heartburn and creates discomfort and other potential risks to a person's health. In this scenario, a person feels or experiences the undigested food or stomach content in the food tube and to the throat. It can damage the inner lining of the tube and of the stomach walls as well.

Acid reflux quickly influences the people having any other health complications. For example, it is common in those with both type 1 and type 2 diabetes. People with asthma may also suffer from acid reflux. Poor digestion problems or other stomach related diseases can also create acid reflux. The treatment of this problem is necessary to be done on time to overcome other health complications, and if not done, then this can cause multiple serious consequences.

According to research, it is shown that acid reflux can be due to improper food intake and consumption of too much fried food and carbonated drinks. This can weaken the power of the stomach to easily digest the food and it can become reactive towards it. Sometimes other health problems can be behind gastric acid reflux. But during the initial stages, with the little concentration of food intake and lifestyle changes, the problem can easily be treated and overcome before it becomes a significant problem.

Treatment of Acid Reflux

Due to poor lifestyle and unhealthy routine, this leads to different health problems, and acid reflux is one of them. Our lives are too much occupied, even that it is hard to find time to eat at the right time. This increases bad food choices and leads to inappropriate meal times. This increases the weight of a person and can lead to obesity. These activities directly impact your sleep and mind activity. When a person does not have a sound mind and feels restless, the digestive system is the most sensitive part of the whole body. This system feels the effects of the stress first.. This leads to inappropriate food digestion and increases acid reflux.

According to the doctors and health advisors, acid reflux is a treatable problem, and with some lifestyle changes, it can be overcome easily. In the treatment of acid reflux, the first thing that matters is diagnosis. In the first recommendation, food that is not allowed to consume includes: fried and fatty food items, processed and canned food, carbonated drinks, alcoholic drinks, citrus, and pepper. These foods can increase the heartburn and restless condition and can create irritation or damage.

Other than the food restriction, it is necessary to reduce the size of the meal that a person consumes in a day. A large meal size can fill the stomach and increase the reaction or irritation. But with smaller meal sizes, the stomach can have a large space and as a result, this reduces the refluxes. As well as it is necessary to take the last meal 3 hours before going to sleep, and do not consume food right before bedtime.

To neutralize the condition, keep your head parallel to the body when you are on the bed. It helps to control the flow of food or acid towards the food canal and offer relieve for heartburn at nighttime. Do not use a high pillow, because it puts exertion or pressure on the stomach and can create a restless condition.

With the lifestyle and dietary changes implemented, keep consulting the doctor and get medication as well. The medication can help to neutralize the impact and prevent the acid reflux from gaining a serious impact on your health.

Complications Due to Acid Reflux

Acid reflux is a digestive related problem that can be treated with the medication and a change in lifestyle. But if not treated properly and if the condition is allowed to go untreated for a long time, then it can affect the stomach and other body parts as well. It is reflux or backflow of stomach acid or food towards the food canal that creates heartburn. Due to the movement of the fluid in the throat, a person may experience irritation and dry cough as well. A person with gastric acid reflux usually feels the pain in the chest that feels like a heart pain, but it is actually due to the gas and the effect of reflux comes from the stomach.

Sometimes the symptoms get worse if not treated on time. Acid reflux can damage the inner lining of the esophagus or can be a reason for bleeding as well. This complication can create a stomach ulcer or can be chronic with time. Due to untreated stomach acid reflux, it is also noticed that some people even face the chronic problem of narrowing of their esophagus lining. With time, it can be the cause of esophageal cancer as well. This severe complication cannot just affect the person's health but also can be the cause of limited activities or reduced productivity. In the worst scenario, these can be life-threatening as well.

The best remedy to avoid such issues is to keep the focus on a small problem and get the proper treatment from the health advisor on time.

If you are at the initial stage or facing the acid reflux, then it is important to pay attention to your activities. With just small change in their diet and lifestyle, a person cannot just overcome the issue but also get the treatment they need on time. Even with natural food and home-based remedies, it is easy to treat and control acid reflux. All you need is to avoid the unhealthy or acidic food choices that increase the acidity in the stomach. Consume the food with minimum spices and salt that reduces the irritation. Also have small meal sizes throughout the day. Furthermore, we have some recipes that will help you to make delicious food that offers relief for acid reflux as well.

Chapter 4:
Recipes for Breakfast

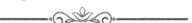

1. Soft & delicious French toast

*Preparation time: 10 minutes l **Cooking time:** 08 minutes l **Servings:** 4*

Ingredients:

- ❖ 4 eggs
- ❖ 8 slices of sandwich bread
- ❖ 1 ½ teaspoons crushed cinnamon
- ❖ ¾ cup milk
- ❖ 1 teaspoon vanilla extract
- ❖ 2 tablespoon ground sugar
- ❖ A pinch of salt
- ❖ 1 tablespoon butter

Directions:

In a bowl, whisk eggs well. Add vanilla extract, salt, and milk. Mix all the ingredients well. Dip the bread slices in the egg mixture. Take another bowl and mix cinnamon and sugar together. Now sprinkle this ground sugar and cinnamon on both sides of the bread. Take a nonstick pan with butter. Heat the butter and cook the egg soaked slices until its color becomes golden brown. Cook it for 3 to 4 minutes per side on a low medium flame. Serve and enjoy.

Nutritional Information:

Carbohydrates 39g, Calories 370, Protein 14g, Fats: 17g, Sugar 9g.

2. Cinnamon & vanilla toast

*Preparation time: 5 minutes l **Cooking time:** 5 minutes l Servings: 2*

Ingredients:

- ❖ 3 eggs
- ❖ 5 slices sandwich bread
- ❖ 1 tablespoon butter
- ❖ 3 tablespoons milk
- ❖ 1 teaspoon vanilla extract
- ❖ A pinch of salt
- ❖ A pinch of sugar
- ❖ ½ teaspoon cinnamon

Directions:

Take a bowl and mix eggs, milk, salt, sugar, cinnamon, and vanilla extract together. Whisk all the ingredients well. Soak the bread slices in the mixture properly. Now take a skillet with the butter and place it over a medium-low flame. Once the butter is melted, place the slices in the skillet one by one to cook. Cook it for around two to three minutes on each sides and it is ready to serve. If you want, you can also serve it with the maple syrup, but this is optional.

Nutritional Information:

Carbohydrates 51g, Calories 422, Protein 8g, Fats: 16g, Sugar 18g.

3. Breakfast frittata

Preparation time: 15 minutes l Cooking time: 15 minutes l Servings: 8

Ingredients:

- ❖ 3 tablespoons chopped onions
- ❖ ¼ cup sliced tomatoes
- ❖ 1 cup cubed boiled potatoes
- ❖ 12 eggs
- ❖ 1 cup ground cooked sausage
- ❖ 2 tablespoons finely chopped parsley
- ❖ 2 tablespoons olive oil
- ❖ ½ cup ground bacon
- ❖ ½ cup grated cheese
- ❖ 1 teaspoon salt
- ❖ ½ teaspoon black pepper

Directions:

Place the oven skillet over a medium flame. Add oil and add potatoes and onion in it and cook for around 5 minutes. Now add tomatoes, sausage, and bacon and cook for a minute. In a bowl, beat the eggs, salt, and black pepper. Now carefully pour the beaten eggs into the pan. Cook it for few minutes and when it's more than half cooked, add cheese and parsley in it. Now put the skillet in the oven to cook it for around 10 minutes in the preheated oven at a temperature of 350F.

Nutritional Information:

Carbohydrates 05g, Calories 268, Protein 16g, Fats: 20g, Sugar 1g.

4. Scrambled egg with veggies

*Preparation time: 5 minutes l **Cooking time**: 10 minutes l **Servings**: 2*

Ingredients:

- ❖ 4 eggs
- ❖ 1 chopped tomatoes
- ❖ ¼ cup milk
- ❖ ½ cup ground green pepper
- ❖ ½ teaspoon salt
- ❖ ¼ cup cubed green onions
- ❖ 1/8 teaspoon black pepper
- ❖ ½ cup grated broccoli
- ❖ ½ cup cubed mushrooms

Directions:

Take a medium-sized mixing bowl and mix egg, milk, green pepper, black pepper, salt, and onion in it. Mix the ingredients well until all the ingredients are well blended. Take a pan and cook the mushrooms and broccoli for around 5 minutes. Add spinach and cook for an additional 2 minutes. Now add the prepared mixture. Now add tomatoes and cook the eggs properly for around 3 to 4 minutes. Transfer it to the serving plate. The scrambled eggs and veggies are ready to serve.

Nutritional Information:

Carbohydrates 9g, Calories 96, Protein 14g, Fats 10g, Sugar 4g.

5. Eggs benedict

*Preparation time: 10 minutes l **Cooking time:** 20 minutes l **Servings:** 4*

Ingredients:

- ❖ 4 eggs
- ❖ 1 tablespoon warm water
- ❖ 4 bacon slices
- ❖ 1 tablespoon butter
- ❖ 1 tablespoon lemon juice
- ❖ 2 split and toasted muffins
- ❖ ½ cup melted butter
- ❖ A pinch salt
- ❖ 2 egg yolks

Directions:

Place water filled pan over the high flame and bring it to boil. Now reduce the flame and break an egg gently in a bowl and gently transfer it to the pan. Cook them for around 3 minutes. Now, with the help of a spatula, transfer the eggs from the pan to a paper towel. In a skillet, melt the butter over a medium-high flame. Now cook bacon in this butter for around 4 minutes. Place the bacon on the first half of the muffin and place cooked eggs on it. To make the sauce, add egg yolks, lemon juice, salt, pepper, and water in a blender and blend it thoroughly. Add hot melted butter and blend it well. Now pour the sauce on the muffins over eggs and serve.

Nutritional Information:

Carbohydrates 29.6g, Calories 879, Protein 31.8g, Fats: 71.1g.

6. Pear banana nut muffins

Preparation time: 5 minutes l Cooking time: 15 minutes l Servings: 12

Ingredients:

- ❖ ½ cup crumbled almonds
- ❖ ½ cup rolled oats
- ❖ 1 peeled and ground pear
- ❖ 2 mashed bananas
- ❖ ¾ cup milk
- ❖ 1 teaspoon cinnamon
- ❖ 2 cups flour
- ❖ ½ cup melted coconut oil
- ❖ 1 teaspoon vanilla

Directions:

Preheat the oven to 360F. Set the 24 muffin cups in a baking tray and prepare them with the baking sheet. Set these cups aside. Now take a big mixing bowl and add all the ingredients in it. Whisk all the ingredients well and pour the mixture in the prepared muffin cups evenly. Bake the muffins for 15 minutes. Check them by inserting a matchstick in the middle and bake the muffins until the match stick comes out clean. At this point, the muffins are ready to serve.

Nutritional Information:

Carbohydrates 13g, Calories 119, Protein 2g, Fats: 6g, Sugar 2g.

7. Blueberry muffins

Preparation time: 10 minutes l Cooking time: 30 minutes l Servings: 12

Ingredients:

- ❖ 2 cups flour
- ❖ 2 eggs
- ❖ ½ cup milk
- ❖ ½ cup butter
- ❖ 2 teaspoons baking powder
- ❖ 2 cups washed and drained blueberries
- ❖ 1 ¼ cups sugar
- ❖ 1 teaspoon vanilla extract
- ❖ ½ teaspoon salt
- ❖ 3 teaspoons sugar

Directions:

In a bowl, mix butter and 1 ½ cup sugar well. Now add eggs and vanilla extract and whisk them well. Now add all the remaining ingredients in this batter and whisk it well until all the ingredients are merged properly. Take a baking dish and set the 12 muffin cups in the baking dish with the muffin liner. Now pour the batter in the prepared cups and sprinkle the sugar on tops. Place the cups in the preheated oven at 375F for around 30 to 35 minutes or until baked well.

Nutritional Information:

Carbohydrates 39g, Calories 252, Protein 4g, Fats: 9g, Sugar 22g.

8. Pumpkin nut muffins

Preparation time: 10 minutes l Cooking time: 10 minutes l Servings: 16

Ingredients:

- ❖ 2 eggs
- ❖ 2 cups flour
- ❖ 1 cup brown sugar
- ❖ ¼ teaspoon cinnamon
- ❖ 1 ½ teaspoons baking powder
- ❖ 1 cup melted butter
- ❖ 1 teaspoon vanilla extract
- ❖ ½ teaspoon salt
- ❖ 1 cup walnuts
- ❖ 15-ounce pumpkin puree
- ❖ ½ teaspoon pumpkin pie spice

Directions:

Set the oven to 375F and set a tray with muffin cups. Prepare the muffin cups with a baking sheet. Take a bowl and mix baking powder, flour, and salt together. Beat the brown sugar and pumpkin puree in a bowl. Combine eggs, vanilla, and melted butter and whisk well. Now add dry ingredients mixture, walnuts, and remaining ingredients and combine them well. Scoop the prepared batter in the muffin cups evenly. Now place it in the preheated oven to cook for around 18 minutes and it is ready to serve.

Nutritional Information:

Carbohydrates 27.7g, Calories 122, Protein 3.1g, Fats: 3.3g, Sugar 18.9g.

9. Egg & vegetable mix muffin

*Preparation time: 20 minutes l **Cooking time**: 30 minutes l **Servings**: 4*

Ingredients:

- ❖ 8 eggs
- ❖ 1 chopped onion
- ❖ 2 minced garlic cloves
- ❖ 2 diced bell peppers
- ❖ 10 sliced mushrooms
- ❖ 2 cups chopped spinach
- ❖ A pinch salt
- ❖ ½ teaspoon ground black pepper
- ❖ 1 tablespoon butter

Directions:

Place the skillet over the medium flame and melt the butter. Stir the garlic, bell peppers, and onion in it and cook for around 5 minutes. Add spinach and mushrooms in it and cook for an additional 3 minutes. Add salt and black pepper in it. In a mixing bowl beat the eggs and add the cooked mixture in it. Take the prepared muffin cups with the baking sheet. Pour the batter in the muffin cups and cook them in the preheated oven for around 20 to 25 minutes.

Nutritional Information:

Carbohydrates 7g, Calories 370, Protein 15g, Fats: 10g.

10. Cauliflower breakfast muffin

*Preparation time: 10 minutes l **Cooking** time: 30 minutes l **Servings**: 6*

Ingredients:

- ❖ 2 eggs
- ❖ 2 ½ cups cubed cauliflower
- ❖ 2 cups shredded cheese
- ❖ 2/3 cup cubed lean ham
- ❖ 1 tablespoon chopped flaxseed
- ❖ 1/8 teaspoon ground black pepper
- ❖ ¼ teaspoon salt

Directions:

Set the oven at a temperature of 375F. Set 12 muffin cups in a tray with the muffin liner. Take a bowl and beat eggs well. Now add all the remaining ingredients in the eggs and whisk well until all the ingredients are merged well. Spoon the prepared batter in the muffin tins and place them in the preheated oven to bake for around 30 minutes. To check whether it is cooked well, take a match stick and insert it in the middle of a muffin cup. If it comes out clean, it means muffins are ready.

Nutritional Information:

Carbohydrates 5g, Calories 214, Protein 15g, Fats: 15g, Sugar 2g.

11. Carrot & apple oat muffin

Preparation time: 15 minutes l *Cooking time: 25 minutes* l ***Servings:*** *12*

Ingredients:

- ❖ 2 eggs
- ❖ ½ cup olive oil
- ❖ ½ cup brown sugar
- ❖ ¾ cup oats
- ❖ ½ cup ground sugar
- ❖ 2 teaspoons vanilla
- ❖ 1 peeled and ground apple
- ❖ ½ cup flour
- ❖ 1 cup grated carrots
- ❖ 1 teaspoon baking powder
- ❖ 1 cup dried cranberry
- ❖ ½ teaspoon salt

Directions:

Prepare the muffin cups with the muffin liner and preheat the oven at the temperature of 350F. In a bowl, beat the eggs, vanilla, oil, and sugar well. Now combine oats, baking powder, salt, and flour together and whisk well. In this mixture, add all the remaining ingredients and combine them well. Now pour the mixture in the muffin tins and bake it for around 30 minutes. Leave them for around 5 minutes to cool down and serve.

Nutritional Information:

Carbohydrates 35g, Calories 281, Protein 11g, Fats: 12g.

12. Breakfast egg muffins

*Preparation time: 5 minutes l **Cooking time**: 20 minutes l **Servings**: 12*

Ingredients:

- ❖ 10 eggs
- ❖ ¼ teaspoon salt
- ❖ ¼ teaspoon ground black pepper
- ❖ 1/3 cup milk
- ❖ 1 tablespoon minced fresh chives
- ❖ 1 cup shredded cheddar cheese
- ❖ 6 oz. cooked bacon

Directions:

Set the oven temperature to 375F. Set the 12 muffin tins in a baking dish and place the muffin liner in it. In a mixing bowl, add milk and eggs and beat them well. Now add ¾ cup cheese, salt, pepper, and cooked bacon and mix all the ingredients well. Spoon the mixture in the prepared muffin tins and sprinkle chives and remaining cheese on it. Bake the muffins in the preheated oven for about 20 minutes. Leave them for a few minutes to cool down and then transfer it to the serving plate.

Nutritional Information:

Carbohydrates 1g, Calories 171, Protein 13g, Fats: 12g.

13. Potato & spinach frittata

*Preparation time: 10 minutes l **Cooking time**: 20 minutes l **Servings**: 6*

Ingredients:

- ❖ 6 eggs
- ❖ 6 sliced potatoes
- ❖ 1/3 cup milk
- ❖ 2 tablespoons olive oil
- ❖ 2 tablespoons cubed onion
- ❖ 1 teaspoon minced garlic
- ❖ ½ cup grated cheese
- ❖ 1 cup roughly chopped spinach
- ❖ 1/8 ground black pepper
- ❖ ½ teaspoon salt

Directions:

Place a skillet with olive oil over a medium flame. Add potatoes, cover and cook it for approximately 10 minutes. Add onions, garlic, salt and pepper, and spinach in it and stir for about 2 minutes. Take a mixing bowl and add milk and egg in it and beat them well. Pour the beaten eggs in the skillet of vegetables and reduce the heat. Now add cheddar cheese, cover it with a lid, and cook it for about 5 to 7 minutes.

Nutritional Information:

Carbohydrates 28g, Calories 281, Protein 12g, Fats: 13g, Sugar 3g.

14. Tomato toast with Ricotta

Preparation time: 5 minutes l Cooking time: 5 minutes l Servings: 4

Ingredients:

- ❖ 2 tablespoons chopped onion
- ❖ 1 cup ricotta cheese
- ❖ 1/8 teaspoon crushed black pepper
- ❖ 3 thickly sliced tomatoes
- ❖ 4 slices of bread
- ❖ ¾ teaspoon Italian seasoning

Directions:

Take a mixing bowl and combine chopped onion, ricotta cheese, black pepper, and Italian seasoning. Mix until all the ingredients are combined well. Now put this mixture aside. Take the bread slices and toast both sides. It's time to assemble the toast. Take the bread slice and spread the prepared mixture on it. Now, place the tomato slices on it. Now your delicious tomato toast with ricotta is ready to serve.

Nutritional Information:

Carbohydrates 41g, Calories 127, Protein 12g, Fats: 10g, Sugar 4g.

15. Avocado & egg toast

Preparation time: 5 minutes l Cooking time: 5 minutes l Servings: -1

Ingredients:

- ❖ 1 egg
- ❖ 1 slice of bread
- ❖ 1 oz. mashed avocado
- ❖ A pinch of salt
- ❖ A pinch of black pepper
- ❖ 1 tablespoon olive oil
- ❖ 1 teaspoon hot sauce

Directions:

In a bowl, add the mashed avocado, salt, and pepper together. Mix it well. Take a small non-stick pan and place it over a medium-low flame. Now pour oil in it and carefully crack the egg in the small pan. Cover the pan with its lid and cook it for few minutes. On the other hand, toast the slice and add the mashed avocado on top. Sprinkle salt and pepper on it and place the cooked egg on top. Pour hot sauce over it and serve. Hot sauce is exceptional, so if you wish to add it, you can add it.

Nutritional Information:

Carbohydrates 23g, Calories 299, Protein 12g, Fats: 10g, Sugar 4g.

16. Yogurt & blueberry smoothie

Preparation time: 5 minutes l Cooking time: 0 minutes l Servings: 3

Ingredients:

- ❖ ½ cup yogurt
- ❖ ¾ cup of coconut water
- ❖ 1 sliced banana
- ❖ 2 ½ cups frozen blueberries
- ❖ 1 tablespoon ground flaxseed
- ❖ 1 cup baby spinach
- ❖ A few coconut flakes
- ❖ ¼ teaspoon vanilla extract

Directions:

Take a blender and combine yogurt, banana, frozen blueberries, spinach, flaxseed, vanilla extract, and coconut water. Blend all the ingredients for about one minute or until the ingredients become the consistency of a smoothie. Add ice in it to chill. If the mixture is thicker and not according to your own desire, add more coconut water or ice to your preference. When the mixture meets your preferred consistency, pour it in the serving glass. Add few coconut flakes as a garnish and serve it immediately.

Nutritional Information:

Carbohydrates 34g, Calories 180, Protein 9g, Fats: 3g, Sugar 21g.

17. Peanut butter & banana smoothie

*Preparation time: 5 minutes l **Cooking time:** 0 l Servings: 2*

Ingredients:

- ❖ 6 tablespoons peanut butter
- ❖ 2 bananas
- ❖ 1/8 teaspoon salt
- ❖ 1/3 cup rolled oats
- ❖ 2 cups of milk
- ❖ 1 tablespoon protein powder
- ❖ 1 teaspoon honey
- ❖ 6-8 ice cubes

Directions:

Add oats in a blender and blend them well until it turns to a powder. Now peel the bananas and slice them. Add the sliced bananas in the blender with all the remaining ingredients. Blend all the ingredients together until combined. Add ice cubes in it and blend it well to chill the smoothie and to reach the required consistency. Add more milk or ice cubes as needed until the smoothie reaches your desired consistency. Now pour it in the serving glass and enjoy.

Nutritional Information:

Carbohydrates 39g, Calories 370, Protein 14g, Fats: 17g, Sugar 9g.

18. Quinoa fruit salad

*Preparation time: 5 minutes l **Cooking time**: 0 l Servings: 4*

Ingredients:

- ❖ 2 cups properly cooked quinoa
- ❖ ½ cup blueberries
- ❖ 1 teaspoon chopped mint leaves
- ❖ 1 cup diced strawberries
- ❖ 1 peeled and cubed mango
- ❖ ½ cup blueberries
- ❖ 2 tablespoons of nuts
- ❖ ¼ cup apple cider vinegar
- ❖ 1 tablespoon sugar
- ❖ ¼ cup olive oil
- ❖ 3 tablespoons lemon juice
- ❖ 1 lemon zest

Directions:

Take a bowl and add vinegar, oil, sugar, lemon juice, and zest in the bowl and mix all the ingredients well. Put this bowl to the side. Now take another bowl and add mango, quinoa, nuts, blueberries, and strawberries. Whisk all the ingredients thoroughly. Now pour the mixed vinegar matter in the quinoa mixture and stir all the ingredients thoroughly. Move it to the serving bowl and garnish it with mint leaves and serve immediately.

Nutritional Information:

Carbohydrates 34g, Calories 308, Protein 4g, Fats: 18g, Sugar 15g.

19. Almonds & nuts with oats

Preparation time: 5 minutes l Cooking time: 1 minute

l Servings: 3

Ingredients:

- ❖ 1 cup almonds
- ❖ 1 cup dried blueberries
- ❖ 3 cups oats
- ❖ 1 cup brown sugar
- ❖ 1 cup walnuts
- ❖ 1 ½ tablespoons cinnamon
- ❖ 1 cup crushed flaxseed
- ❖ ½ tablespoon salt
- ❖ 2 cups of milk

Directions:

In a blender, blend one cup of oats, brown sugar, salt, almonds, and cinnamon. Blend all these ingredients thoroughly. Transfer the blended ingredients into a bowl. Now, add the remaining ingredients in the bowl and prepare the mixture and mix it well. Now, store the mixture in a bowl with a lid. Before serving it, add ¾ cup milk in the ½ cup prepared mixture and microwave it in a bowl for around one minute. Add the milk at the time of serving. You can also use water or almond milk instead of milk.

Nutritional Information:

Carbohydrates 53g, Calories 355, Protein 9g, Fats: 13g, Sugar 19g.

20. Quinoa & chia porridge

*Preparation time: 5 minutes l **Cooking time**: 20 minutes l **Servings**: 1*

Ingredients:

- ❖ ¼ cup quinoa
- ❖ ½ cup of water
- ❖ ½ cup milk
- ❖ 1 tablespoon chia seed
- ❖ ¼ teaspoon ground cinnamon

Directions:

Take a pan and add milk and water in it and place it over a medium-high flame. When it comes to a boil, add quinoa, cinnamon and chia seeds and mix well. Now, reduce the heat and cover the pan with the lid. Cook it over a medium-low flame for around 12 to 15 minutes. Stir it frequently and cook it until the liquid is fully absorbed. When the quinoa starts to appear, remove it from the stove and set it aside for around 5 to 10 minutes to cool it down. After 5 minutes, serve it and if you want, you can top it with fruits, nuts, or milk.

Nutritional Information:

Carbohydrates 51g, Calories 356, Protein 14g, Fats: 11g, Sugar 8g.

21. Peanut butter and banana pudding with chia seeds

*Preparation time: 5 minutes l **Chilling time:** 4 hours l Servings: 4*

Ingredients:

- ❖ 1 cup almond milk
- ❖ 1/2 cup yogurt
- ❖ ½ cup peanut butter
- ❖ 2 tablespoons honey
- ❖ ½ cup chia seeds
- ❖ 1 teaspoon vanilla extract
- ❖ 1 sliced banana
- ❖ 1 tablespoon roasted peanut

Directions:

Take a mixing bowl and combine the yogurt and butter and mix them well. Now, add vanilla extract, honey, chia seeds, and almond milk. Mix all the ingredients well until they become smooth. Pour the prepared mixture in a container and refrigerate it for at least 4 hours. After four hours, scoop the pudding in the serving bowl and garnish it with the banana slices and roasted peanuts. Now it is ready to serve.

Nutritional Information:

Carbohydrates 34g, Calories 403, Protein 14g, Fats: 25g, Sugar 18g.

22. Banana zucchini oatmeal cups

*Preparation time: 15 minutes l **Cooking time**: 25 minutes l **Servings**: 15*

Ingredients:

- ❖ 2 cups grated zucchini
- ❖ ¼ cup maple syrup
- ❖ 3 small mashed bananas
- ❖ 3 cups oats
- ❖ ½ cup almond milk
- ❖ 1 tablespoon crushed flaxseed
- ❖ 1 teaspoon vanilla extract
- ❖ 1 teaspoon cinnamon
- ❖ 1 tablespoon baking powder
- ❖ ¼ teaspoon salt
- ❖ 3 tablespoons water

Directions:

Prepare the muffin tins with a muffin liner. Set the temperature of the oven to 375F. In a small bowl, mix flax and water and set it aside. In another bowl, combine the mashed bananas, almond milk, zucchini, maple syrup, and the prepared flax mixture. Stir all the ingredients well. Add the remaining ingredients in it and mix it thoroughly. Now, pour the prepared mixture in the muffin tins and bake it in the preheated oven for around 23 to 25 minutes.

Nutritional Information:

Carbohydrates 26g, Calories 215, Protein 5g, Fats: 3g, Sugar 9g.

23. Slow cooker sausages & egg casserole

*Preparation time: 30 minutes l **Cooking time:** 06-08 hours l **Servings:** 10*

Ingredients:

- ❖ 12 eggs
- ❖ ¼ teaspoon garlic powder
- ❖ 16 ounces cooked and crumbled sausages
- ❖ 32 ounces grated frozen hash browns
- ❖ ½ teaspoon black pepper
- ❖ 1 teaspoon salt
- ❖ ¼ cup milk
- ❖ 6 chopped onions
- ❖ 12 ounces grated cheddar cheese

Directions:

Take a 6-quart slow cooker, and with the cooking spray, grease its insert. Now place the first layer of half hash browns in the cooker and sprinkle the salt and pepper. Now place the second layer of half sausages, then half onions and grated cheese. Repeat the layers in the same sequence and finish it by topping with cheese. Take a mixing bowl and mix eggs, salt, pepper, garlic powder, and milk. Whisk it well and pour it over the top layer. Cook for around 4 to 6 hours in the slow cooker over low heat.

Nutritional Information:

Carbohydrates 17g, Calories 431, Protein 24g, Fats: 29g.

24. Cauliflower chaffle

Preparation time: 5 minutes l Cooking time: 5 minutes l Servings: 2

Ingredients:

- ❖ 1 egg
- ❖ 1 cup rice cauliflower
- ❖ ½ cup grated parmesan cheese
- ❖ ½ cup grated mozzarella cheese
- ❖ ¼ teaspoon crushed black pepper
- ❖ ¼ teaspoon garlic powder
- ❖ ¼ teaspoon salt
- ❖ ½ teaspoon Italian seasoning

Directions:

Mix all the ingredients, reserving 1/8 cup of parmesan cheese, into a blender and blend well. Now take a waffle maker and sprinkle the grated remaining parmesan cheese in it. Cover the waffle bottom with the cheese properly. Now fill the waffle maker with the prepared blended mixture. Now cover its top with the remaining cheese properly. Cook it for approximately 4 to 5 minutes or cook it until it becomes crispy and its color changes to a golden color. Make 4 mini chaffles with this batter and serve immediately.

Nutritional Information:

Carbohydrates 7g, Calories 246, Protein 20g, Fats: 16g, Sugar 2g.

25. Garlic parmesan chaffle

*Preparation time: 5 minutes l **Cooking time:** 15 minutes l **Servings:** 2*

Ingredients:

- ❖ 1 egg
- ❖ 1/8 teaspoon Italian seasoning
- ❖ ¾ teaspoon coconut flour
- ❖ ¼ teaspoon garlic powder
- ❖ 1 tablespoon parmesan cheese
- ❖ 1 tablespoon melted butter
- ❖ ¼ teaspoon basil seasoning
- ❖ 1 cup grated mozzarella cheese
- ❖ A pinch of salt
- ❖ ¼ teaspoon baking powder

Directions:

Preheat the oven to 400F temperature. Let the waffle maker get hot and grease it. Take a bowl and add eggs, half the mozzarella cheese, Parmesan cheese, flour, baking powder, Italian seasoning, and salt in it and stir all the ingredients well. Now scoop half of the prepared batter on the waffle maker and close it. Cook it for about 4 minutes. When it is cooked, remove it from the waffle and place it on a plate. In a bowl, mix the melted butter and garlic powder. Cut the cooked muffins into two pieces and brush the prepared garlic butter on its top. Place them in a baking pan and top it with the remaining mozzarella cheese. Bake it in the preheated oven for around 4 to 5 minutes. Remove it from the oven and before serving, sprinkle basil on top.

Nutritional Information:

Carbohydrates 3g, Calories 270, Protein 16g, Fats: 21g, Sugar 1g.

26. Jalapeno & bacon chaffle

Preparation time: 5 minutes *l Cooking time:* 5 minutes *l Servings:* 5

Ingredients:

- ❖ 3 eggs
- ❖ 4 slices bacon
- ❖ 3 tablespoons coconut flour
- ❖ 8-ounces cream cheese
- ❖ 3 washed, dried and de-seeded jalapeno peppers
- ❖ ¼ teaspoon salt
- ❖ 1 teaspoon baking powder
- ❖ 1 cup grated cheese

Directions:

Take a pan and cook bacon over medium heat until it becomes crispy. In a bowl, mix salt, baking powder. and flour. In another bowl, beat cream cheese well. Preheat a greased waffle maker. Whisk eggs in another bowl and add half cream cheese and grated cheese. Add mixed dry ingredients and mix them well. In the end, mix jalapeno into the mixture. Scoop the batter into the waffle maker and cook it over medium heat for around 5 minutes. Transfer it to the serving plate and pour the remaining cream on it and serve.

Nutritional Information:

Carbohydrates 5g, Calories 509, Protein 23g, Fats: 45g.

27. Chaffle garlic sticks

*Preparation time: 3 minutes l **Cooking time:** 11 minutes l **Servings:** 2*

Ingredients:

- ❖ 1 egg
- ❖ 1 tablespoon butter
- ❖ 1 cup grated Mozzarella cheese
- ❖ ½ teaspoon garlic powder
- ❖ ½ teaspoon basil
- ❖ 1 tablespoon almond flour

Directions:

Preheat the waffle maker. Take a mixing bowl combine egg, ¼ teaspoon garlic powder, ½ teaspoon basil, flour, and half cup Mozzarella cheese in it and mix it well. Add the half batter in the maker and cook for around 4 minutes. Cook the rest of the batter in the same way. Take another bowl and mix butter, remaining garlic powder. Microwave it for around 30 seconds. Now take a baking sheet and place the waffles on it. With the help of a brush spread the garlic butter on the waffle. Sprinkle cheese on the waffles and bake it for around 1 or 2 minutes at the 400 degrees' temperature or until the cheese melted.

Nutritional Information:

Carbohydrates 2g, Calories 231, Protein 13g, Fats: 19g, Sugar 1g.

28. Avocado cucumber smoothie

Preparation time: 5 minutes | Cooking time: 0 |
Servings: 1

Ingredients:

- ❖ 1 avocado
- ❖ 1 teaspoon lemon juice
- ❖ 1 cup almond milk
- ❖ ½ cucumber
- ❖ 1 apple
- ❖ ¼ cup stalk celery
- ❖ ½ tablespoon ground dill

Directions:

Take the avocado and remove its stone. Dice and cut the celery and cucumber. Cut the apple into small cubes. Take a blender and put all the ingredients in it. Blend all the ingredients well until combined. If the consistency of smoothie is thicker, add more milk to it. When you reach your preferred consistency, transfer it to the serving glass. If you want the cold smoothie, then add ice cubes in it while blending.

Nutritional Information:

Carbohydrates 21g, Calories 339, Protein 5g, Fats: 17g, Sugar 3g.

29. Sweet potato spinach bowl

Preparation time: 10 minutes l Cooking time: 15 minutes l Servings: 01

Ingredients:

- ❖ ½ peeled, diced, sweet potatoes
- ❖ ½ diced avocado
- ❖ ¼ cup chopped fresh spinach
- ❖ ½ cup quinoa
- ❖ ¼ cup ground walnuts
- ❖ ¼ cup olive oil
- ❖ ¼ cup vinegar
- ❖ 3 teaspoons Dijon mustard

Directions:

For the dressing, in a mixing bowl, add oil, Dijon mustard, and vinegar. Mix all these ingredients well and set it aside. Cook the quinoa according to the instructions given on the pack. Now take another medium-sized mixing bowl. Add quinoa, spinach, walnuts, sweet potato, and avocado in this mixing bowl. Mix all the ingredients properly. Now pour the prepared dressing on it and it is ready to serve.

Nutritional Information:

Carbohydrates 42g, Calories 285, Protein 9g, Fats: 11g.

30. Mexican bean & avocado toast

Preparation time: 20 minutes l Cooking time: 10 minutes l Servings: 4

Ingredients:

- ❖ 1 ½ cup diced tomatoes
- ❖ 4 tablespoons olive oil
- ❖ 2 minced garlic cloves
- ❖ 1 teaspoon lemon juice
- ❖ 1 sliced avocado
- ❖ 1 teaspoon ground cumin
- ❖ 2 cans drained black beans
- ❖ 1 chopped bunch coriander
- ❖ 1 chopped onion
- ❖ 1 teaspoon chili flakes
- ❖ 4 slices of bread

Directions:

In a bowl, add ¼ onion, oil, and lemon juice. Mix these ingredients well. Place a skillet over a medium flame and fry the remaining onion in the oil. Add garlic and cook for an additional 1 minute. Now add chili flakes and cumin and cook for a few seconds. Now add beans and ¼ cup water, whisk it well and cook it. Add tomato and cook for an additional 1 minute. Season the cooked material with the coriander. Now, with the remaining oil, toast the bread. Place the toast on a serving plate and top it with the cooked batter. Serve it immediately.

Nutritional Information:

Carbohydrates 30g, Calories 368, Protein 12g, Fats: 19g, Sugar 6g.

Chapter 5:
Recipes for Lunch

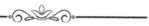

1. Vegan green bean casserole

Preparation time: 10 minutes l Cooking time: 20 minutes l Servings: 4

<u>Ingredients</u>

- ❖ Green beans – 1 pound, cut in half
- ❖ Sea salt – to taste
- ❖ Shallot – 1, medium, minced
- ❖ Garlic – 2 cloves, minces
- ❖ Mushrooms – 1 cup, chopped
- ❖ Flour – 2 tablespoons
- ❖ Black pepper – to taste
- ❖ Butter – 2 tablespoons
- ❖ Vegetable broth – ¾ cup
- ❖ Almond milk (unsweetened) – 1 cup
- ❖ Fried onion – 1 ½ cup, divided

Directions

Preheat the oven to 204 C or 400F. Take a large pot and bring water to boil. Add salt while water is boiling. Add green beans to the boiling water, allow it to boil for at least 5 minutes; drain and wash with cold water. Then drain the green beans properly and set them aside. Take a skillet, preferably oven-safe, heat the butter in it and put garlic and shallot. When the shallot starts to become translucent, add salt and pepper, and stir continuously. When the shallot is completely translucent, add finely chopped mushrooms to skillet and cook for another 4 to 5 minutes until the mushrooms become brown and cooked. Now add flour to the skillet and stir so it can combine well. Add vegetable broth slowly and whisk so the flour does not form any lumps in the liquid. Add almond milk and let it simmer. When it starts to simmer, reduce the heat to low and allow it to reduce until it reaches your desired thickness, or for about 7 minutes. When you reach the desired consistency, remove the skillet from heat and add 1/3 of fried onions and green beans. Toss until well combined. Sprinkle the rest of the fried onions on top. Bake the skillet for at least 15 minutes and heat in the oven until the top turns brown. Serve instantly!

2. Roasted vegetables

*Preparation time: 15 minutes l **Cooking time**: 40 minutes l **Servings**: 2*

Ingredients

- ❖ Butternut squash – 1, small, cubed
- ❖ Sweet potato – 1, cubed
- ❖ Yukon gold potatoes – 3, cubed
- ❖ Olive oil – ¼ cup
- ❖ Balsamic vinegar – 2 tablespoons
- ❖ Salt – to taste
- ❖ Red Bell pepper – 2, diced
- ❖ Red onion – 1, quartered
- ❖ Fresh thyme – 1 tablespoon
- ❖ Fresh rosemary – 2 tablespoons
- ❖ Black pepper – to taste

Directions

Preheat the oven at 245C or 475F. Take a large bowl and add red bell pepper, butternut squash, sweet potatoes, red onion and Yukon gold potatoes. Take a small bowl and combine rosemary, thyme, balsamic vinegar, olive oil, black pepper, and salt. Add this mixture to the large bowl of vegetables; toss well so the mixture can combine with the vegetables evenly. Take a roasting pan, brush with oil, and spread the vegetables on it evenly. Put the pan into the preheated oven and roast for at least 40 minutes or until the vegetables are properly cooked. Stir after every 10 minutes. Serve warm!

3. Cauliflower stuffing

*Preparation time: 15 minutes l **Cooking time:** 40 minutes l **Servings:** 6*

Ingredients

- ❖ Onion – 1, chopped
- ❖ Celery stalks – 2, chopped
- ❖ Cauliflower – 1 small, chopped
- ❖ Mushrooms – 1 cup, chopped
- ❖ Rosemary – 2 tablespoons, chopped
- ❖ Sage – 1 tablespoon, freshly chopped
- ❖ Butter – 4 tablespoons
- ❖ Carrot – 2, large, peeled, chopped
- ❖ Black pepper – grounded, to taste
- ❖ Parsley – ¼ cup, chopped
- ❖ Chicken broth – ½ cup

Directions

Take a large pan or skillet, melt the butter over medium heat, add celery, onion and carrot, and cook for 8 minutes until soft. Add mushrooms and cauliflower and freshly grounded black pepper and salt, then cook for 10 minutes until tender. Now add rosemary, parsley and sage and stir well. Add chicken broth to the skillet and cook for 10 minutes until the liquid is absorbed by the vegetables. Serve warm!

4. Chicken lettuce wraps

*Preparation time: 30 minutes l **Cooking time:** 20 minutes l **Servings:** 4*

Ingredients

- ❖ Hoisin sauce – 5 tablespoons
- ❖ Soy sauce – 2 tablespoons
- ❖ Rice vinegar – 2 tablespoons
- ❖ Sesame oil – 1 teaspoon
- ❖ Turkey – 1 pound
- ❖ Garlic – 3 cloves, minced
- ❖ Ginger – 1 tablespoon, freshly minced
- ❖ Scallions – ½ cup, thin sliced, divided
- ❖ Cornstarch – 1 teaspoon
- ❖ Vegetable oil – 2 teaspoons, divided
- ❖ Mushrooms – 8 ounces, chopped
- ❖ Onion, carrots, bell pepper – diced (Optional)
- ❖ Chestnuts – 1 can, finely chopped
- ❖ Butter lettuce – 2 heads, small
- ❖ Hot sauce, red pepper flakes – for garnish

Directions

Take a small bowl, combine hoisin sauce, rice vinegar, soy sauce and sesame oil. For a thicker sauce, you can add cornstarch. Take a large pan or skillet, heat the oil at a medium temperature, put the turkey into the pan and cook for 8 to 10 minutes until cooked and the pink color of the meat vanishes; set aside. In the same pan, heat the oil, add the vegetables (optional ones) and mushrooms, and stir and cook for 5 minutes until tender. Stir in ginger, chestnuts and garlic; cook for about a minute until fragrant. Add the cooked turkey into the pan and add half of the scallions; combine well. Now add the sauce into the pan and cook for another minute until it bubbles. Separate the leaves of lettuce from its branch and pile them. Put the chicken material into each leaf. Garnish with scallions, red pepper flakes and hot sauce according to your taste.

5. Zucchini sushi

Preparation time: 20 minutes l Cooking time: 20 minutes l Servings: 2

Ingredients

- ❖ Zucchini – 2, medium
- ❖ Crab meat – 1 can
- ❖ Carrot – ½ thinly cut
- ❖ Avocado – ½ unit, diced
- ❖ Cucumber – ½ unit, thinly cut
- ❖ Cream cheese – 4 oz.
- ❖ Hot sauce – 1 teaspoon
- ❖ Lime juice – 1 teaspoon
- ❖ Sesame seeds – 1 tablespoon, toasted

Directions

With the help of a vegetable peeler, thinly slice the zucchini in flat strips; put the stripes on a paper towel to sit. Take a medium bowl, whisk hot sauce, cream cheese and lime juice; set aside. Take 2 strips of zucchini, spread the cream cheese mixture on top, add pinch of avocado, crab, carrot and cucumber and roll it. Repeat with the rest of the strips. Sprinkle sesame seeds on top before serving.

6. Avocado, beans and chicken salad

Preparation time: 13 minutes l Cooking time: 7 minutes l Servings: 4

Ingredients

- ❖ Olive oil – 3 tablespoons
- ❖ Chili powder – 1 tablespoon
- ❖ Garlic – 4 cloves, minced
- ❖ Black beans – 1 can, rinsed
- ❖ Salt – to taste
- ❖ Green onion – 2 units, sliced
- ❖ Avocado – 2, diced
- ❖ Cilantro – 1/3 cup
- ❖ Cayenne pepper – 1 pinch
- ❖ Boneless chicken breast – 1.25 pound – diced
- ❖ Cumin 1 tablespoon
- ❖ Black pepper – to taste
- ❖ Cherry tomatoes – 2 cups, halved
- ❖ Lime juice – 4 tablespoons
- ❖ Apple cider vinegar – 2 tablespoons
- ❖ Honey – 3 tablespoons

Directions

Take a large skillet and heat olive oil at medium heat. Add chicken, chili powder, and cumin. Cook for about 5 minutes until done. Add garlic and cook for another minute until fragrant. Add the beans, black pepper, and salt. Stir well until combined. Transfer the mixture into a large bowl. Add green onions, tomatoes, avocado, apple cider vinegar, cilantro and lime juice; stir and combine. Add the cayenne, honey and remaining salt and pepper;. Your meal is ready to be served.

7. Avocado stuffed shrimp salad

*Preparation time: 10 minutes l **Cooking time:** 15 minutes l **Servings:** 4*

Ingredients

- ❖ Cooked Shrimps – ½ pound, chopped
- ❖ Celery – ½ cup
- ❖ Parsley – 1 tablespoon
- ❖ Dijon Mustard – 2 teaspoons
- ❖ Lemon juice – 1 ½ teaspoons
- ❖ Tarragon – ¾ teaspoon, dried
- ❖ Onion – ¼ cup, chopped
- ❖ Mayonnaise – 3 tablespoons
- ❖ Capers – 4 teaspoons, drained
- ❖ Seasoned salt – ¼ teaspoon
- ❖ Pepper – 1/8 teaspoon
- ❖ Avocado – 2 medium unit, halved

Directions

In a bowl, combine shrimp, onion, celery, mayonnaise, parsley, capers, Dijon mustard, salt, pepper, lemon juice and tarragon. Take the avocado and fill this mixture in the center. Serve immediately!

8. Fajita steak salad bowl

Preparation time: 10 minutes | Cooking time: 15 minutes | Servings: 4

Ingredients

- ❖ Lettuce – 7 ounces
- ❖ Steak of your choice – 1 lb.
- ❖ Olive oil – 4 tablespoons, divided
- ❖ Bell pepper – 2 cups, strips
- ❖ Corn tortillas – 2
- ❖ Mexican crema sauce – ½ cup
- ❖ Lime juice – 2 tablespoons
- ❖ Chili powder – 2 tablespoons
- ❖ Cumin – 1 teaspoon, grounded
- ❖ Smoked paprika – 1 teaspoon
- ❖ Onion powder – 1 teaspoon
- ❖ Garlic powder – 1 teaspoon
- ❖ Red onion – ½, sliced
- ❖ Corn – 1
- ❖ Black olives – ¼ cup
- ❖ Cherry tomatoes – 4, halved
- ❖ Fresh cilantro – ½ cup

- ❖ Fajita seasoning – ¼ tablespoon
- ❖ Salt – 1 teaspoon, divided
- ❖ Sugar – 1 teaspoon
- ❖ Oregano – ½ teaspoon
- ❖ Cayenne pepper – ½ teaspoon
- ❖ Black pepper – ½ teaspoon
- ❖ Cilantro & jalapenos – for garnish

Directions

Take tortilla and cut it in half. Then cut it into strips almost about ¼ inch of width. Take a large skillet and heat the olive oil on high heat. Add the strips and fry for few minutes, flip and cook until golden brown; drain the oil and dry with paper towel. Season with salt.

In a blender, add chili powder, cumin, paprika, onion powder, garlic powder, sugar, oregano, cayenne pepper, salt and black pepper; blend to combine. Now your fajita seasoning is ready.

Take food processor, add Mexican Crema Sauce, lime juice, cilantro, previously prepared fajita seasoning, and a pinch of salt; process to make a smooth dressing for the salad. Pat dry the steak and apply a generous amount of fajita seasoning on both sides. Take the same skillet and heat the oil on high flame; put steak in the hot oil and cook for 3 minutes from each side; remove from the skillet and let the steak rest for at least 10 minutes. Wipe the remains from the skillet and heat another tablespoon of olive oil; put onion, sear for a minute at high flame, remove from pan. Repeat this process with the peppers. Take the corn cob and flame it over on the flame to get the kernels until charred and popped. Layer the lettuce in a large salad bowl; slice the prepared steak into strips and arrange it with salad, olives, pepper and onions, corm, tortilla strips and the rest. Top your salad with the dressing Garnish with jalapenos and cilantro.

9. Grilled chicken with asparagus & white beans

*Preparation time: 10 minutes l **Cooking time:** 15 minutes l **Servings:** 4*

Ingredients

- ❖ Chicken breast - 4
- ❖ Asparagus – 12 stalks
- ❖ Oil – 1 tablespoon
- ❖ Cannellini beans – 800 g
- ❖ Salt & pepper – 1 teaspoon
- ❖ Garlic – 2 cloves
- ❖ Parsley – ½ cup
- ❖ Olive oil – ½ cup
- ❖ Lemon juice – ¼ cup
- ❖ Dijon mustard – 1 teaspoon

Directions

Apply olive oil on both sides of the chicken and sprinkle salt over it. Take a frying pan and heat the heat a tablespoon of oil; cook chicken in it for 5 minutes from each side until tender. In a pot, boil water with a pinch of water; add asparagus and let it boil until tender; drain. In a small bowl, combine cannellini beans with garlic, onion and parsley. Now add lemon juice, oil, Dijon mustard, pepper and salt in the bean bowl and combine. Slice the chicken; serve with the white bean salad and boiled asparagus.

10. Cardamom chicken with lime leaves

Preparation time: 30 minutes l Cooking time: 1 Hour 15 minutes l Servings: 4

Ingredients

- ❖ Rapeseed – 2 tablespoons
- ❖ Onion – 1, chopped
- ❖ Ginger – 2 tablespoons, grated
- ❖ Garlic – 4 cloves, grated
- ❖ Cardamom pods – 12, lightly crushed
- ❖ Red chili – 1, halved
- ❖ Tomatoes – 400g, chopped
- ❖ Mango chutney – 1 tablespoon
- ❖ Vegetable bouillon powder – 3 teaspoons, divided
- ❖ Basmati rice – 125g
- ❖ Red lentils – 100g
- ❖ Cloves – 4
- ❖ Cinnamon stick – 1
- ❖ Turmeric – 3 teaspoons, halved

- ❖ White pepper – 1 ½ teaspoons
- ❖ Coriander – 1 teaspoon, grounded
- ❖ Cumin – 1 teaspoon
- ❖ Auvergne – 1, cubed
- ❖ Lime leaves – 4
- ❖ Boneless chicken – 1kg
- ❖ Green pepper – 1, sliced
- ❖ Cumin seeds – 1 teaspoon

Directions

Take a large pan and heat the oil; add onion and cook it for 5 minutes until translucent. Put garlic, cardamom, ginger, cinnamon and cloves in the pan; cook for another 5 minutes. Add the rest of the spices into the pan, tomatoes, mango chutney, water and bouillon. Now add Auvergne into the pan; boil the mixture, then let it simmer for at least 15 minutes. Add lime leaves and chicken into the pan, cover it and allow it to cook for at least 40 minutes. After the chicken is cooked, remove the chicken from the pan, shred it into medium pieces, and return it to the pan again. In a saucepan, add 750ml of water, boil the rice along with red lentils, cumin seeds, turmeric and bouillon powder; cover and allow it to cook for at least 20 minutes until rice is tender. Turn off the heat and leave it until the moisture absorbs. Serve the rice with the chicken curry!

11. Chicken Caesar wraps

Preparation time: 15 minutes | Cooking time: 0 minutes | Servings: 6

Ingredients

- ❖ Caesar salad dressing – ¾ cup
- ❖ Parmesan cheese – ¼ cup, grated
- ❖ Garlic powder – ½ teaspoon
- ❖ Cooked chicken breast – 3 cups
- ❖ Torn romaine – 2 cups
- ❖ Caesar salad croutons – ¾ cup, chopped
- ❖ Whole wheat tortillas – 6

Directions

Take a large bowl. Combine dressing, garlic powder, cheese and pepper. Add romaine, chicken and croutons. Take a tortilla, spread over 2/3 cup of the mixture and roll it up. Serve fresh!

12. Sweet potato with broccoli & white beans

*Preparation time: 15 minutes l **Cooking time:** 15 minutes l Servings: 4*

Ingredients

- ❖ Organic broccoli – 8 cups, chopped
- ❖ Garlic – 3 cloves, minced
- ❖ Sweet potato – 1 medium
- ❖ Vegetable broth – 2 cups
- ❖ Paprika – ½ teaspoon
- ❖ Yeast – 1/3 cup
- ❖ White beans – 1 ½ cup
- ❖ Onion – 1, chopped
- ❖ Black pepper – ¾ teaspoon
- ❖ Salt – ¼ teaspoon
- ❖ Bay leaf – 1 leaf
- ❖ Cooked pasta 1 cup (optional)

Directions

In a large pot, bring the water to boil. Add sweet potato and let it boil for 6 minutes until tender. Add broccoli and let it boil for another 3 minutes. After exactly 10 minutes, drain the water away. Place 2/3 of the broccoli in a blender and set aside the rest. Add ½ the sweet potatoes in the blender and set aside the rest. Add half chopped onion into the blender; add yeast, beans, salt, pepper, broth, paprika and garlic. Blend the ingredients well until you get a thick and smooth consistency. Pour this mixture into a pot. Add the rest of the vegetables and bay leaf; boil the mixture and reduce the heat and let it simmer for 5 minutes. If you are using pasta, than do not cook it for long the mixture as it will get mushy. Serve the soup hot!

13. Salmon pasta with lemon

Preparation time: *5 minutes l* **Cooking time**: *20 minutes l* **Servings**: *4*

Ingredients

- ❖ Salmon – 1 pound, boneless
- ❖ Garlic – 2 cloves, sliced
- ❖ Unsalted butter – 4 tablespoons
- ❖ Olive oil – 1 tablespoon
- ❖ Lemon wedges – for garnish
- ❖ Lemon juice – 3 tablespoons
- ❖ Salt – to taste
- ❖ Black Pepper – to taste
- ❖ Pasta of your choice – ½ lb.
- ❖ Parsley – ¼ cup

Directions

Preheat the oven to 199C or 390F. Pat dry the salmon with a paper towel and place it on a baking dish. Apply black pepper and salt all over the fillet; top with garlic slices, olive oil and lemon juice. Bake the fillet for about 15 minutes until done. Take out the dish from the oven and allow it to cool; flake out the fillet into a bit larger pieces (it will break while tossing). Take a medium pan and cook pasta along with parsley; you can also add dill if you like. When the pasta is done, drain it and add salmon chunks along with the juice; toss well to combine. Add more lemon juice if desired. Season with black pepper, salt and lemon wedges. Serve readily!

14. Roasted tomato soup

Preparation time: 20 minutes l Cooking time: 50 minutes l Servings: 4-6

Ingredients

- ❖ Tomatoes - 2 ½ pound
- ❖ Garlic – 5 cloves, peeled
- ❖ Yellow onion – 2, sliced
- ❖ Olive oil – ½ cup
- ❖ Heavy cream – ¾ cup (Optional)
- ❖ Basil leaves – ½ cup, chopped (Optional)
- ❖ Black pepper – to taste
- ❖ Salt – to taste
- ❖ Chick stock – 1 quart
- ❖ Bay leaves – 2
- ❖ Butter – 4 tablespoons
- ❖ Vine cherry tomato – for garnish (optional)

Directions

Preheat the oven at 232C or 450F. Cut the tomatoes in half and put them on a baking tray along with onion slices and garlic clove; if you are using tomatoes for garnishing, then put them to the side as well. Shower the extra virgin olive oil, black pepper and salt all over the tomatoes. Put the tray in the oven and allow it to bake for at least 30 minutes until the tomatoes are caramelized. Separate the tomatoes you put for the garnish and transfer the rest of the material into a pot. Add chicken stock, remaining butter and bay leaves into the pot; cook until starts boil, simmer for at least 20 minutes until reduced to a third at low heat. Add basil leaves (if using); remove bay leaves and add the remaining puree into the blender to make a smooth soup texture. Again, transfer the soup into the pot and heat at low flame; add heavy cream (if using) and get your required consistency (use more chicken stock if required). Serve with the roasted tomatoes, grounded black pepper, salt and a splash of heavy cream on top.

15. Green peas and lentil soup

Preparation time: 10 minutes l Cooking time: 40 minutes l Servings: 4

Ingredients

- ❖ Green lentils – 350 grams
- ❖ Green peas – 350 grams
- ❖ Shallot – 120 grams
- ❖ Carrots – 3 oz.
- ❖ Garlic – 1 clove
- ❖ Salt – to taste
- ❖ Cheese – 4 tablespoons
- ❖ Vegetable broth – 2 liters
- ❖ Olive oil – 10 tablespoons
- ❖ Parsley – 1 bunch
- ❖ Black peppercorn – to taste

Directions

Soak the lentils in water for at least 10 minutes. Take a pan or a pot, heat 3 tablespoons of olive oil and stir fry shallot, garlic and carrots. When the shallot turns translucent, add the green peas and lentils; cook for 5 minutes than add vegetable broth and bring to boil. Once the broth gets to boiling point, reduce the heat, cover the pot and let it simmer until get soup for at least 40 minutes or so. When the soup is ready add black peppercorn and salt to taste. Serve with the topping of parsley, Parmigiano Reggiano Cheese (or cheese of your choice) with olive oil. Serve hot!

16. Grilled chicken salad sandwich

Preparation time: 15 minutes / Cooking time: 15 minutes / Servings: 4

Ingredients

- ❖ Mayonnaise – 1 cup
- ❖ Black pepper – 1/8 teaspoon
- ❖ Garlic powder – 1/8 teaspoon
- ❖ Celery salt – 1/8 teaspoon
- ❖ Grilled chicken – 4 cups
- ❖ Tomato – 1, sliced
- ❖ Celery stalks – 2, sliced
- ❖ Dried cranberries – ½ cup
- ❖ Cashews – 2/3 cup
- ❖ Bread slice – 8, toasted
- ❖ Lettuce – 4 leaves

Directions

In a bowl, combine mayonnaise, garlic powder, black pepper and celery salt. Add cranberries, chicken, celery and cashews in the same bowl and combine until a mixture formed. Apply the mayonnaise mixture on the toasted bread slice; place lettuce and tomato slice; sandwich with the other bread slice.

17. Vegetable barley soup

Preparation time: 5 minutes l Cooking time: 50 minutes l Servings: 6

Ingredients

- ❖ Yellow onion – 1
- ❖ Garlic – 2 cloves
- ❖ Olive oil – 2 tablespoons
- ❖ Carrot – 4
- ❖ Tomato – 1 can, diced
- ❖ Barley – 1 cup
- ❖ Peas – ½ cup
- ❖ Lemon juice – 1 tablespoon
- ❖ Basil – ½ teaspoon, dried
- ❖ Oregano – ½ teaspoon, dried
- ❖ Black pepper – to taste
- ❖ Vegetable broth – 6 cups
- ❖ Russet potato – 1
- ❖ Green beans = 1 cup
- ❖ Corn – ½ cup
- ❖ Parsley – 1 handful, for garnish

Directions

In a pot, heat olive oil; dice garlic and onion on medium heat for around 5 minutes until translucent. Add carrots, tomatoes, basil, barley, oregano, vegetable broth and black pepper; cook for few minutes until the mixture starts to boil; reduce the heat to medium low and let the soup simmer for at least 30 minutes; stir occasionally. Meanwhile, peel and dice the potato into cubes. Check for the barley if it's cooked, then add potatoes into the pot and let it cook for another 10 minutes until tender. Add corn, green beans and peas into the pot; cook for another 5 minutes until well combined. In the end, add lemon juice, adjust the pepper and salt according to your taste. Serve hot with parsley garnished on top!

18. Parmesan Brussels sprouts

Preparation time: 10 minutes l Cooking time: 45 minutes l Servings: 4

Ingredients

- ❖ Brussels sprouts – 12 ounces, halved
- ❖ Olive oil – 2 tablespoons
- ❖ Salt – to taste
- ❖ Black pepper – to taste
- ❖ Parmesan – 1 cup, shredded
- ❖ Cooking spray

Directions

Preheat the oven at 218C or 425F; place a cast-iron skillet in the oven as well. In a medium bowl, toss Brussels sprouts with salt, olive oil and black pepper; add parmesan in the end. Remove the skillet from the oven carefully, spray the cooking oil generously. Spread the Brussels sprouts in the skillet; put back the skillet into the oven and aloe it to bake for about 25 minutes until the Brussels sprouts are brown and tender. Serve warm!

19. Chicken steak soup

*Preparation time: 5 minutes l **Cooking time:** 40 minutes l **Servings:** 6*

Ingredients

- ❖ Butter – 2 tablespoons
- ❖ Vegetable oil – 2 tablespoons
- ❖ Chicken steak – 1 ½ pound
- ❖ Onion – ½ cup, chopped
- ❖ All-purpose flour – 3 tablespoons
- ❖ Paprika – 1 tablespoon
- ❖ Celery – 1 ½ cup, chopped
- ❖ Tomato paste – 1 can
- ❖ Corn – 1 can, drained
- ❖ Carrot – 1 ½ cup, sliced
- ❖ Salt – 1 teaspoon
- ❖ Black pepper – ¼ teaspoon, grounded
- ❖ Chicken broth – 4 cups
- ❖ Water 1 cup
- ❖ Parsley – ½ cup, chopped
- ❖ Celery leaves – 3 tablespoons, chopped
- ❖ Bay leaf – 1

- ❖ Marjoram – ½ teaspoon, dried
- ❖ Yukon gold potato – 1 ½ cup, diced

Directions

Take a skillet and melt the butter on medium heat; stir the steak pieces in the butter along with onions. Cook for 10 minutes until browned. Meanwhile, in a small bowl, combine flour, salt, paprika and black pepper; sprinkle it over the chicken steak pieces and coat well. Take a large pot for soup, add broth, parsley, water, celery leaves, marjoram and bay leaf; add the steak mixture as well; boil the mixture and stir in intervals. When the mixture starts to boil, reduce the flame and let it simmer for about 30 minutes until tender. Add carrots, potato, celery, tomato paste and the corn in the soup let it simmer for another 15 minutes until tender. Remove the bay leaf before serving

20. Lemon garlic shrimp

Preparation time: 5 minutes l Cooking time: 15 minutes l Servings: 4

Ingredients

- ❖ Butter – 2 tablespoons, divided
- ❖ Olive oil – 1 tablespoon
- ❖ Shrimp – 1 lb., deveined
- ❖ Lemon – 1, sliced
- ❖ Lemon juice – 1 tablespoon
- ❖ Garlic – 3 cloves, minced
- ❖ Red pepper flakes – 1 teaspoon, crushed
- ❖ Kosher salt – to taste
- ❖ Dry white wine – 2 tablespoons
- ❖ Parsley – ½ cup, chopped, for garnish

Directions

Take a large skillet and melt butter and olive oil over medium heat; stir shrimp for a minute; add garlic, lemon slices and red pepper flakes along with salt. Cook for about 3 minutes per side until shrimp tenders. Once the shrimp turns pink, remove the skillet from heat; add remaining butter, white wine and lemon juice. Garnish with chopped parsley and sprinkle some salt before serving.

21. Shrimp cucumber bites

Preparation time: 20 minutes | Cooking time: 30 minutes | Servings: 6

Ingredients

- ❖ Olive oil – 1/3 cup
- ❖ Lime juice – 4 tablespoons, divided
- ❖ Honey – 2 tablespoons
- ❖ Garlic – 2 cloves, minced
- ❖ Cilantro – 2 tablespoons, for garnish
- ❖ Cucumber – 2, thick sliced
- ❖ Cajun seasoning – 1 teaspoon
- ❖ Kosher salt – to taste
- ❖ Shrimp – 1 lb., deveined
- ❖ Avocados – 2
- ❖ Red onion – ½ minced
- ❖ Jalapeno – 1, chopped

Directions

Take a large bowl, combine lime juice, olive oil, honey, Cajun seasoning, salt and garlic. Add shrimp in the bowl, coat well and refrigerate for about 30 minutes or more. Take a large skillet. On a medium heat cook the shrimp until tender. It will not take more than 2 minutes or so. Remove the skillet from the heat. Take another bowl and mash avocados, add red onion, lime juice, cilantro, salt and jalapeno. Take a cucumber slice, spread the avocado spread (guacamole) over each slice; place shrimp on top and garnish with cilantro.

22. Balsamic glazed shrimp with quinoa

*Preparation time: 15 minutes l **Cooking time**: 25 minutes l **Servings**: 4*

Ingredients

- ❖ Quinoa – 1 cup
- ❖ Parsley – 1 cup, divided
- ❖ Shrimp – 1 lb., deveined
- ❖ Olive oil – 3 tablespoons, divided
- ❖ Kosher salt – to taste
- ❖ Dry white wine – ½ cup
- ❖ Sugar – 2 tablespoons
- ❖ Black pepper – to taste
- ❖ Garlic – 2 cloves, minced
- ❖ Orange juice – 2 cups
- ❖ Orange zest – 1 tablespoon
- ❖ Lemon juice – 1 tablespoon
- ❖ Balsamic vinegar – 2 tablespoons

Directions

Preheat the oven to 400F. Take a medium pot and prepare quinoa by following the directions given on the box. Sprinkle parsley over the cooked quinoa and set it aside. Pat dry the shrimp, put olive oil, black pepper and salt over them evenly. Take a baking tray, place the shrimp evenly and bake them for about 9 minutes until turned pink. Take a large skillet, heat the olive oil on medium low flame. Add garlic, black pepper, salt, orange zest, balsamic vinegar, lemon juice, orange juice, white wine and sugar. Increase the flame and cook until it boils; when it starts to boil, lower the heat a bit and let the sauce simmer for about 10 minutes until reduced. Take out the shrimp from the oven and toss it in the balsamic sauce. Serve with quinoa and garnish with parsley.

23. Vegetarian chickpea sandwich

Preparation time: 20 minutes l Cooking time: 0 minutes l Servings: 4

Ingredients

- ❖ Chickpeas – 1 can, rinsed
- ❖ Celery – 1 stalk, chopped
- ❖ Onion – ½, chopped
- ❖ Mayonnaise – 1 tablespoon
- ❖ Bread – 8 slices
- ❖ Lemon juice – 1 tablespoon
- ❖ Dill weed – 1 teaspoon, dried
- ❖ Salt – to taste
- ❖ Pepper – to taste

Directions

Take a medium bowl, put drained and rinsed chickpeas in it and mash them with a help of a fork. Add lemon juice, celery, mayonnaise, onion, salt, dill and pepper; mix well to form a mixture. Spread this mixture on the bread slice and sandwich it with another slice.

24. California chicken avocado wrap

*Preparation time: 15 minutes l **Cooking time**: 8 minutes l **Servings**: 4*

Ingredients

- ❖ Turkey bacon – 8 slices
- ❖ Chicken – 2 cups, shredded
- ❖ Salt – to taste
- ❖ Pepper – to taste
- ❖ Mango – 1, chopped
- ❖ Mayonnaise – 6 tablespoons, divided
- ❖ Lime juice – 2 tablespoons
- ❖ Avocado – 1 large
- ❖ Whole wheat tortillas – 4
- ❖ Romaine – 2 cups, shredded
- ❖ Tomato – 1, diced

Directions

Take a large skillet and cook turkey bacon strips until crispy; set aside in paper towel plate. Take a large bowl, combine shredded chicken, black pepper, salt, mayonnaise, mango and lime juice. In another bowl, peel the avocado and mash; add the remaining mayonnaise, black pepper and salt; mix well and set aside. Take a tortilla, spread the avocado mixture over it leaving an inch boarder; put the lettuce, 2 turkey bacon slices and tomato. Spread the chicken mixture over the veggies; roll up the tortilla like a burrito. Cut each of the rolled-up tortilla in half before serving.

25. Baked eggs in avocado

Preparation time: 10 minutes l Cooking time: 15 minutes l Servings: 6

Ingredients

- ❖ Avocado – 2, halved
- ❖ Egg – 6
- ❖ Black pepper and salt – to taste
- ❖ Chives – 2 tablespoons, freshly chopped

Directions

Preheat the oven at 213C or 425F. Take a baking tray and coat it with generous amount of cooking spray. Scoop out some avocado from the mid of each halved unit to make space. Crack 1 egg gently inside the space of the avocado; season with black pepper and salt. Place the avocados in the oven and bake them for around 15 minutes until the egg white sets. Garnish with chives and serve immediately.

26. Skillet steak with corn salad

Preparation time: 10 minutes | Cooking time: 30 minutes | Servings: 4

Ingredients

- ❖ Boneless beef steak – 1 pound, strips
- ❖ Onion – 1, wedges
- ❖ Thyme – ½ teaspoon, dried
- ❖ Canola oil – 2 tablespoons
- ❖ Beef broth – ¾ cup
- ❖ Tomatoes – 1 can, diced
- ❖ Corn – 2 cans, drained
- ❖ Cooked rice – for serving

Directions

Take a large skillet, heat the oil, cook beefsteaks along with thyme and onion on medium heat for about 15 minutes until pinkish color disappears. Drain out the excess water; add wine and let it simmer for about 10 minutes until the liquid evaporates completely. Stir the diced tomatoes and again let it simmer for 15 minutes. Add the corn in the last and let it heat a bit. Serve with cooked rice!

27. Chicken stir fry

*Preparation time: 30 minutes l **Cooking time**: 35 minutes l **Servings**: 6*

Ingredients

- ❖ White rice – 2 cups
- ❖ Water – 4 cups
- ❖ Soy sauce – 2/3 cup
- ❖ Brown sugar – ¼ cup
- ❖ Cornstarch – 1 tablespoon
- ❖ Ginger – 1 tablespoon, freshly minced
- ❖ Garlic – 1 tablespoon, minced
- ❖ Red pepper flakes – ¼ teaspoon
- ❖ Chicken breast – 3, boneless, sliced
- ❖ Sesame oil – 2 tablespoons, divided
- ❖ Bell pepper – 1, sliced
- ❖ Water chestnuts – 2 can, sliced
- ❖ Broccoli – 1 head, broken
- ❖ Carrots – 1 cup, sliced
- ❖ Onion – 1, large chunks

Directions

In a saucepan, boil water along with rice; reduce the heat to low, cover and allow to simmer until the water evaporates the from rice, for about 25 minutes. In a small bowl, combine brown sugar, soy sauce and corn starch; add garlic, ginger and red pepper and mix. Marinate the chicken with the sauce and refrigerate for at least 15 minutes. Take a skillet and heat the sesame oil over medium high heat; stir the water chestnuts, bell pepper, carrots, broccoli and onion until tender; remove these vegetables from skillet and set aside. Take out the chicken and save the marinate. Heat the sesame oil and cook chicken in the skillet on medium high heat until the pink color disappears, almost 3 minutes per side. When the chicken is half cooked, return the vegetables into the pan along with the reserved marinate material. Boil the material and cook for 7 minutes until the chicken is properly done. Serve with rice!

28. Pasta with broccoli and tomato sauce

Preparation time: 10 minutes l Cooking time: 20 minutes l Servings: 2

Ingredients

- ❖ Pasta – 6 oz.
- ❖ Broccoli – ½ lb.
- ❖ Garlic – 2 cloves, chopped
- ❖ Shallot – 1, chopped
- ❖ Capers – 1 tablespoon
- ❖ Calabrian Chile pasta - 1 ½ teaspoon
- ❖ Parmesan cheese – ¼ cup, grated
- ❖ Tomato paste – 2 tablespoons
- ❖ Mascarpone cheese – 2 tablespoons

Directions

In a pot, boil water with a pinch of salt. Meanwhile, cut the broccoli head into ½ inches. Put the pasta in the boiling water and cook for 5 minutes. After 5 minutes, put broccoli in the pot as well and allow it to boil until tender for around another 5 minutes. Reserve ½ cup of the boiling water and drain the rest. In a medium pan heat the olive oil on medium heat; add shallot, garlic and capers; stir for a minute until translucent; add Chile paste and tomato paste. Allow to cook for 2 minutes, stir continuously. Add the ½ cup of reserved water into the pan and cook for another 2 minutes until thickened. Add salt and black pepper to taste. Remove the sauce from heat. Add cooked broccoli, pasta and mascarpone. Combine and heat for another 2 minutes so the pasta can coat completely. Serve with garnished Parmesan cheese.

29. Salmon with lemon and dill

Preparation time: 10 minutes | Cooking time: 25 minutes | Servings: 2

Ingredients

- ❖ Salmon – 1 pound
- ❖ Butter – ¼ cup
- ❖ Lemon juice – 5 tablespoons
- ❖ Dill weed – 1 tablespoon, dried
- ❖ Garlic powder – ¼ teaspoon
- ❖ Salt – to taste
- ❖ Black pepper – to taste

Directions

Preheat the oven to 175C or 350F. Grease the baking dish with oil. In a small bowl, combine butter and lemon juice; place the salmon fillets into the baking tray and drizzle over the butter mixture onto it; season garlic powder, dill, pepper and salt all over the fillet. Place the dish into the oven and bake for about 25 minutes until salmon is flaked with the help of fork. Serve hot!

30. Barbeque halibut steak

Preparation time: 10 minutes l Cooking time: 15 minutes l Servings: 2

Ingredients

- ❖ Halibut steak – 1 pound
- ❖ Butter – 2 tablespoons
- ❖ Brown sugar – 2 tablespoons
- ❖ Garlic – 2 cloves, minced
- ❖ Soy sauce – 2 teaspoons
- ❖ Black pepper – ½ teaspoon, grounded
- ❖ Lemon juice – 1 tablespoon

Directions

Preheat the barbeque grill at medium high heat. In a small saucepan, add brown sugar, butter, garlic, soy sauce, lemon juice and pepper; heat the pan over medium heat until sugar dissolves; stir occasionally. Oil the grill, Brush the brown sugar sauce on to the halibut steak and place them on the grill; cook each side for about 5 minutes until done. Serve hot!

Chapter 6:
Recipes for Dinner

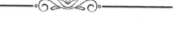

1. Mushroom and Veggie Soup

Preparation time: 20 minutes | Cooking time: 30 minutes | Servings: 5-6 persons

Ingredients:

- ❖ 3 tbsp. Olive/vegetable oil
- ❖ 8 cups vegetable sodium broth
- ❖ 1 diced yellow onion
- ❖ 12 ounces trimmed and chopped mushrooms
- ❖ Minced garlic cloves
- ❖ 2 cups florets of broccoli
- ❖ 1 diced zucchini
- ❖ 1/4 cup Soy sauce
- ❖ 1 tsp dried thyme
- ❖ 1 tsp oregano
- ❖ 3-4 bay leaves
- ❖ Optional to enhance flavor- 1 tbsp apple cider vinegar

Directions:

In a stockpot, add up oil and onion in it. Sauté the onion for a good amount of time, about 7 minutes, until it has turned soft while maintaining to stir recurrently. Now add garlic to the pot and sauté it till it turns aromatic. Add mushrooms, zucchini, thyme, bay leaves, vegetable broth, broccoli, soy sauce, and oregano and simmer the mixture until good lot of 15 minutes. Add salt and vinegar for appeasing and enhancing flavor, depending on your preference.

2. Potato and Almond Soup

*Preparation time: 30 minutes l **Cooking time**: 30 minutes l **Servings**: 4-5 cups/ 2-4 persons*

Ingredients:

- ❖ 2 medium sized potato
- ❖ 2 tbsp. virgin olive oil
- ❖ 4 garlic cloves
- ❖ 2 cups water
- ❖ 1 onion
- ❖ 1 cup blanched almonds
- ❖ Kosher salt (sea salt)
- ❖ 2 tbsp. apple cider vinegar
- ❖ 2 thyme
- ❖ Grounded black pepper

Directions:

Set the oven to 450 degrees to preheat it, and line the baking tray with aluminum foil. Take peeled potatoes in a bowl and chop them into chunks. In a similar manner, peel onions and chop them to chunk size. Next, peel the garlic cloves and chop them coarsely. Place both the elements in the bowl alongside the potatoes and drizzle oil over the mixture before spreading in on the baking tray/sheet. Let the mixture be roasted for a good lot of 15 to 20 minutes so that it turns out to be tender. Bring almonds to simmer in a pot and let it be cooked for 2 straight minutes before combining it and the roasted batter in a blender. Add salt, thyme and black pepper over to brighten up the flavor as required.

3. Red Lentil Salsa Soup

Preparation time: 10-15 minutes | Cooking time: 30-45 minutes | Servings: 9 cups/6 persons

Ingredients:

- ❖ 1 tbsp. Olive oil
- ❖ 2 medium sized diced onions
- ❖ 3 Diced carrots
- ❖ 3 Minced cloves of garlic
- ❖ 3 tsp Cumin
- ❖ 3 tsp Oregano dried
- ❖ Broth (vegetable or chicken - 4 cups)
- ❖ 3 cups water
- ❖ 1.5-2 cups green lentils, dried
- ❖ 2 cups salsa

Directions:

Heat oil in a stockpot and add onions and carrots to it. Stir the mixture for about 7 minutes, until it becomes tender. Sauté garlic, oregano, and cumin while repetitively whipping it for total of 30 seconds. Insert water, broth, salsa, and lentils into the heated pot and bring it to boil proceeded by simmering it until lentils become soft. Garnish thyme and parsley over the soup and to brighten up your taste. Voila! Bon appetite!

4. Garlic pasta with roasted Brussels sprouts and tomatoes

*Preparation time: 10 minutes l **Cooking time**: 35-40 minutes l **Servings**: 7-8 cups/4 persons*

Ingredients:

- ❖ 15 Fairly sliced Brussels sprouts
- ❖ 5-6 sun dried tomatoes
- ❖ 30 grape or datterini tomatoes
- ❖ ¼ sliced shallot
- ❖ 1 garlic clove
- ❖ 10 basic leaves
- ❖ 1 tsp olive oil
- ❖ Salt (as per requirement)
- ❖ 11 oz spaghetti
- ❖ ½ cup Fairly grated Reggiano cheese

Directions:

Set the oven to preheat at 425F. Cover the baking tray with tomatoes, Brussels sprouts and garlic while drizzling it with oil and a pinch of salt and set it in the oven. Let the mixture be baked for about 30 minutes. During this time, boil the pasta in a utensil. Sauté shallots in a skillet for about 4 minutes and if preferred, introduce anchovies in it to brighten up the flavor. Now add the roasted mixture in the pan along with the pasta. Toss and enjoy.

5. Sun-dried tomato pesto pasta

*Preparation time: 10 minutes l **Cooking time:** 15-20 minutes l **Servings:** 4*

Ingredients:

- ❖ 12 ounces Penne pasta
- ❖ 1 cup/freshly packed Basil leaves
- ❖ 2 Cloves of garlic
- ❖ 1/2 cup finely shredded Parmesan
- ❖ 1 Sun dried tomato in an olive oil jar
- ❖ Ground black pepper and salt

Directions:

Bring the pasta to be boiled in a pot and set it aside after draining 3/4th of the liquid. On the other hand, place sun-dried tomatoes along with garlic, oil, pepper and salt in a blender and blend it intermittently until the tomatoes get fairly slashed. Now add up the blended mixture in a skillet and toss it with Parmesan cheese. Introduce pasta into the pan, toss it and enjoy the eternal flavor.

6. Creamy Tuscan Chicken

Preparation time: 10 *minutes l **Cooking time:*** 15 *minutes l **Servings:*** 6

Ingredients:

- ❖ 2 tbsp. Olive oil
- ❖ 1/2 cup Parmesan cheese
- ❖ Skinless/1.5 pounds sliced chicken breasts
- ❖ 1 cup Chopped spinach
- ❖ 1 cup heavy cream
- ❖ 1/2-1 cup sun-dried tomatoes
- ❖ 1-2 tsp garlic powder
- ❖ 1 tsp Italian seasoning

Directions:

In a large pot, cook chicken for a good time of 10 to 15 minutes until each of the side has properly been cooked and turned brown. Set the cooked chicken aside, introduce broth (chicken), Parmesan cheese, heavy cream and Italian seasoning in a skillet and toss it until the batter starts to condense. Place sun-dried tomatoes along with spinach and let the mixture simmer so that the spinach gets sagged. Mix chicken with the paste and add few pinches of garlic powder to enhance the flavor.

7. Chicken thigh with garlic and rosemary

Preparation time: 5 minutes l Cooking time: 30 minutes l Servings: 4 persons

Ingredients:

- ❖ Skinless/6 Chicken bone-in thighs
- ❖ 4 minced cloves of garlic
- ❖ 4 tbsp. olive oil
- ❖ Ground pepper and salt (as required)
- ❖ 3 tbsp. fresh rosemary
- ❖ 1 cup grape tomatoes

Directions:

Place skinless chicken in a skillet and toss it with salt and pepper. Now after setting the chicken aside, add garlic and rosemary in a heated skillet containing olive oil and stir it for good amount of 1 minute until it turns aromatic. Introduce chicken into the pan while tossing it for 10 minutes and just before it is about to be cooked, add sun-dried tomatoes while whisking it for about 5 to 10 minutes. Serve chicken with rice or pasta depending on your choice and enjoy the delicious food.

8. One-pot beef with broccoli

*Preparation time: 20 minutes l **Cooking time:** 25 minutes l **Servings:** 6 persons*

Ingredients:

- ❖ 2 pounds of beef
- ❖ 4 tsp corn starch
- ❖ 1.5 cup hot water
- ❖ 2 tbsp. brown sugar
- ❖ 4 cup broccoli
- ❖ Olive oil and salt (as required)
- ❖ 4 tbsp. soy sauce
- ❖ 3 cloves of garlic
- ❖ 2 tbsp. sesame oil

Directions:

Place all the liquid sauces in a mixing bowl and mix it thoroughly. Cook beef in a pan until it turns brown and when cooked, add the mixture of sauce into it. Bring the mixture to simmer while adding the vegetables into the skillet. Just when the vegetables and the beef turn tender, serve the dish alongside rice and enjoy the meal.

9. Vegan chickpea shakshuka

Preparation time: 5 minutes l Cooking time: 25 minutes l Servings: 2 persons

Ingredients:

- ❖ 2 tbsp. olive oil
- ❖ 1 onion
- ❖ 1 bell pepper
- ❖ 400 grams/1 sliced tomato
- ❖ 2 cloves of garlic
- ❖ 2 tbsp. tomato paste
- ❖ canned/400gram/1 cooked chickpeas
- ❖ Canned olives
- ❖ Salt, basil leaves, thyme (as required)
- ❖ Black pepper, rosemary, chili powder (to taste)

Directions:

Add the chopped vegetables, i.e. onion, bell peppers and cloves of garlic, into a heated pan. Sauté the added ingredients for at least 5-6 minutes until it turns soft and translucent. Introduce sun-dried tomatoes along with the tomato paste and the mentioned spices (rosemary, thyme, chili powder, salt) by bringing the mixture to be seethed. Add the dried chickpeas to the prepared sauce and stir it for 20 straight minutes so that it absorbs the flavor. Add olives to the pan and basil leaves for garnishing. Bon appetite!

10. Steak with lemon mashed potatoes

*Preparation time: 10 minutes l **Cooking time**: 20 minutes **Servings**: 4 people*

Ingredients:

- ❖ 1-1.5 pounds Yukon potatoes
- ❖ 2-3 tbsp. olive oil
- ❖ 1 cup frozen peas
- ❖ 2 tbsp./2 tsp respectively lemon juice and zest
- ❖ 2 sliced shallots
- ❖ Unsalted/1-1.5 tbsp. Butter
- ❖ 1-2 pounds/2 strips each thickening about ¾ strips of chicken/beef steak
- ❖ Salt and pepper (to taste)

Directions:

Set the oven to 450F to preheat it. Now introduce the gold, peeled potatoes into the pot along with a cold water. Let the potato be boiled for about 15 minutes and just before it has been cooked, add peas to the pot in the final 5 minutes. After draining the liquid from the pot, add lemon zest and juice to it and mash it finely. On the other hand, cook the steak to your desired wellness and set it aside. To prepare the sauce, add sliced shallots into the skillet and transfer butter, salt and pepper, including wine to enhance the flavor to your preference. Serve the mashed potato with the respective prepared sauce and steak. Now enjoy

11. Easy baked chicken for heartburn

*Preparation time: 15 minutes l **Cooking time**: 45-50 minutes l **Servings**: 4 persons*

Ingredients:

- ❖ Skinless/4 Chicken breasts
- ❖ 4 tbsp. olive oil
- ❖ 3 tbsp. shredded Parmesan cheese
- ❖ Salt and ground black pepper (to taste)
- ❖ 1 cup bread crumbs
- ❖ Italian seasoning (to taste)

Directions:

Set the oven to 400F. In a mixture bowl, add shredded Parmesan cheese along with bread crumbs and the spices to coat the chicken breast. Pat the chicken breasts with traces of olive oil and introduce it into the prepared concoction of bread crumbs. Line up the patted, coated chicken breasts on the baking tray and set it aside to be baked for about 40 minutes. Bon appetite!

12. Chickpeas Hummus

Preparation time: 10 minutes *l Cooking time:* 10 minutes *l Servings:* 1.5 cups/6 people

Ingredients:

- ❖ 1 cup chickpeas, canned or cooked
- ❖ 1/4 cup lemon juice
- ❖ 1 minced garlic
- ❖ 1/2 tsp cumin
- ❖ 2 tbsp. olive oil
- ❖ 3 tbsp. water
- ❖ Tahini and salt (to taste)

Directions:

In a blender or a food processor, add tahini paste and the cup of chickpeas. Once blended for 1 minute, add olive oil, salt, and water along with cumin and minced garlic to the processor and blend it for another good 5 minutes. Add chickpeas into the blender and process it for about 2 minutes. To maintain the consistency, add water into the hummus until it reaches the desired texture.

13. Banana sorbet

*Preparation time: 5 minutes l **Cooking time**: 0 minutes l **Servings**: 1 person*

Ingredients:

- ❖ 1 ripe bananas
- ❖ ½ tbsp. chocolate chips
- ❖ 1 tbsp. caramel syrup

Directions:

Once you pare banana a day before you have to prepare the sorbet, carve it down and store it in freezer. The very next day, grab the frozen, sliced bananas and introduce it in the blender along with any other ingredient (chocolate chips, caramel syrup, thawed chocolate) of your choice. Blend it and enjoy the moment all yourself or freeze it for consuming it later on.

14. Chicken with butternut squash

Preparation time: 30 minutes l Cooking time: 30 minutes l Servings: 2-4 persons

Ingredients:

- ❖ 4-6 tbsp. butter
- ❖ 1 tsp cloves of garlic crumbled
- ❖ 1 lb. or pound butternut squash cut into cubes
- ❖ 1/4 cup whole flour
- ❖ 4 ounces green beans
- ❖ Skinless, boneless/1 pound chicken breasts
- ❖ 1 tsp paprika
- ❖ Oregano, salt (to taste)

Directions:

Set the oven to be preheated at about 400F. Cover the baking tray with a sheet of aluminum foil or parchment. Now, in order to prepare butternut squash, cut the top portion of it while holding its base and cutting it into fine 2 pieces. Use a peeler to scrape off the covering from the butternut squash. Remove the seeds within and cut it into slices. When done, combine all the other ingredients along with the butternut squash and skinless chicken breasts. Toss the spices in it and place it down on the baking sheet. Set it aside to be baked for around 1 hour. Increase the heat in the oven to 450 degree Fahrenheit so that the chicken gets perfectly cooked inside and out. For brightening up the flavor, add thyme, oregano and paprika over and serve it hot.

15. Grilled pesto chicken

*Preparation time: 60 minutes l **Cooking time:** 30 minutes l **Servings:** 4-6 persons*

Ingredients:

- ❖ 1 cup pesto
- ❖ 1 tsp sugar
- ❖ 1/4 cup Vinegar
- ❖ 1 tsp salt
- ❖ Skinless, boneless/2 pounds chicken breasts

Directions:

To marinate the chicken effectively and evenly, take a ziplock bag and place the boneless/skinless chicken breast in it along with vinegar, pesto, sugar and salt inside. Shake it thoroughly so that the chicken breasts get marinated consistently. Set the zip locked bag aside in a refrigerator for about 2 hours. Now, to grill the chicken breast, preheat the oven or the open-air grate and place the marinated chicken upon it so that it gets equally cooked on both sides for good lot of 10 to 15 minutes. To let the chicken, absorb the flavor, let it sit aside for 5 minutes before shredding it on. Meanwhile, if one wants to cook it indoors, a skilled or a non-stick pan can be utilized to prepare the savory dish.

16. Bake potato & bacon

Preparation time: 30 minutes |Cooking time: 14 minutes l Servings: 4

Ingredients:

- ❖ 4 Idaho potatoes
- ❖ Salt and black pepper to taste
- ❖ 2 tablespoons of extra virgin olive oil

For filling:

- ❖ 6-8 pieces of bacon
- ❖ 2 green onions finely chopped
- ❖ ½ cup sour cream
- ❖ 1 cup shredded cheddar cheese
- ❖ 1 cup shredded cheddar cheese

Directions:

First of all, preheat the oven to 375F. Cook the bacon until golden and crisp out, cut it into small pieces and set aside until you are ready to use it. Wash the potatoes well to scrub all dust and dry them well before seasoning them, then poke the potatoes with a knife at 6 to 7 different places so filled steam will not allow them to burst. Drizzle potatoes with 2 tablespoons of the extra-virgin olive oil and season with salt and pepper to taste then bake them in the oven for 60 to 90 minutes. After baking mash, the opening of potatoes with a fork and fill it with cheese and bake again for 10 minutes until cheese gets melted. Garnish it with onions, sour cream and bacon. Enjoy!

17. Red onion chicken with rice

Preparation time: 60 minutes | Cooking time: 35 minutes | servings: 4

Ingredients:

- ❖ 1 pinch black pepper
- ❖ 1 tbsp. sunflower oil
- ❖ 2 boneless chicken breast
- ❖ 300 ml water
- ❖ 1 tbsp. fresh coriander
- ❖ 1 cinnamon stick
- ❖ 2 tbsp. curry powder
- ❖ 1 tbsp. raisin
- ❖ 85g frozen peas
- ❖ 4 tbsp. low fat natural yogurt
- ❖ 1 large red onion
- ❖ 100g basmati rice
- ❖ 1 tbsp. fresh mint
- ❖ 1 pinch salt

Directions:

Preheat the oven to 190F. Brush oil over the chicken and pepper it with curry powder. After tossing the onion slices in a roasting tin, add chicken over it and place it into the oven to cook for 30 minutes. Meanwhile, crisp onion separately in a pan. Boil rice in water until tender by adding 1 cinnamon stick and a pinch of salt and add peas to cook for 10 to 12 minutes. To serve, place rice on plate, add chicken, and sprinkle the onions as a topping. Add mint and coriander and serve with yogurt.

18. Bean and chicken sausages stew

Preparation time: 20 minutes | Cooking time: 20 minutes |Servings: 5

Ingredients:

- ❖ 2 tbsp. olive
- ❖ 1½ tsp sweet smoked paprika
- ❖ 3 chopped garlic cloves
- ❖ 2 chopped celery
- ❖ 1 chopped onion
- ❖ 1 ½ Kg chopped tomatoes
- ❖ 1 Yellow capsicum.
- ❖ 1 chicken stock cube
- ❖ 1 Red capsicum
- ❖ 400g can of beans
- ❖ 6 cooking sausages
- ❖ 1 tbsp. fresh coriander

Directions

Have oil in a pan and fry onions for 5 minutes, then add all chopped vegies yellow and red capsicum, celery sticks and cook for 5 minutes. Then add sausages to fry for 5 more minutes. After that, add chicken and water and cook for 10 minutes. Add garlic, smoked paprika, and cumin to cook until all aromas came out. Add tomato paste and thyme, then add chicken cubes and stir it, now keep it on the stove for 40 minutes. Afterwards, add beans and cook for more 5 minutes. Then season with black pepper. Now serve.

19. Brown sugar meatloaf

Preparation time: 10 - 15 minutes | Cooking time: 90 minutes | Servings: 5

Ingredients:

- ❖ ½ cup packed brown sugar
- ❖ 1½ pounds lean ground beef
- ❖ ½ cup ketchup
- ❖ ¾ cup milk
- ❖ 2 eggs
- ❖ 1 ½ teaspoons salt
- ❖ ¼ teaspoon ground black pepper
- ❖ 1 small onion
- ❖ ¼ teaspoon ground ginger
- ❖ ¾ cup cracker crumbs

Directions:

Let preheat oven at 350 degrees. Brush the oil over the loaf pan. Now add beef sprinkle brown sugar, pour ketchup and toss well. In a separate bowl ass milk, eggs, salt, black pepper, ginger, and make a fine blend. Apply the mixture over beef evenly. Toss the beef into cracker crumb and set in pan. Sprinkle onion and bake it for 80 to 85 minutes or until cooked and juicy. Enjoy with ketchup or a sauce of your choice.

20. Cocktail Meatballs

Preparation time: 15 minutes | *Cooking time: 90 minutes* | *Servings: 5*

Ingredients:

- ❖ 1 pound lean ground beef
- ❖ 2 tablespoons water
- ❖ 1 egg
- ❖ 3 tablespoons crushed onion
- ❖ ½ cup bread crumbs

Directions:

Preheat oven at 375 degrees for 20 minutes. In a mixing bowl, add all ingredients beef, egg, water, bread crumbs and onions. Mix them well and take a small quantity with spoon and make round balls. Take a baking pan and set parchment paper with oil grease. Set the meat round balls into the baking try and bake for 20 to 25 minutes or until cooked and turned brown. Serve with sauce, ketchup or anything you love. Enjoy!

21. Grilled corn cob with lime

Preparation time: 15 minutes |*Cooking time: 25 minutes* | *Servings: 4*

Ingredients:

- ❖ ½ cup butter
- ❖ 1 can chipotle peppers
- ❖ 1 zest lime
- ❖ Salt to taste
- ❖ 4 corns sticks

Directions:

Take a grill and heat at a low medium flame. Grease it with oil. Take a bowl and add butter, chipotle peppers, lime zest, and salt and mix until combine. Let the mixture set aside for few minutes. Now toss the mixture over the corncobs and let them grill for 20 to 25 minutes until it cooked well. Every 10 minutes, change the side of corncobs over the grill. Serve immediately!

22. Mexican baked fish

Preparation time: 20 minutes | *Cooking time:* 15 minutes | *Servings:* 5

Ingredients:

- ❖ 1 cup of salsa
- ❖ ½ cup crushed corn chips
- ❖ 1 ½ shredded cheddar cheese
- ❖ ¼ cup sour cream
- ❖ 1 ½ cup avocado
- ❖ 1 ½ pound cod
- ❖ 2 fish fillets

Directions:

Preheat oven to 400 degrees and set the baking tray by greasing it and setting it aside. Put the fish fillets on baking tray and sprinkle shredded cheese, corn chips and salsa over it. Remember, the topping must be with corn chips. Put into oven and bake for 15 to 20 minutes or until cooked. Now remove and add avocado slices and bake for more 5 minutes. Now serve with sour cream.

23. Sesame noodles with chicken

Preparation time: 5 minutes | Cooking time: 20 minutes | Servings: 5

Ingredients:

- ❖ 1 pack of spaghetti
- ❖ 3 tbsp. sesame oil
- ❖ 2 scallions
- ❖ 2 tsp. ginger paste
- ❖ 1 tbsp. garlic paste
- ❖ 1 tsp. brown sugar
- ❖ 2 tbsp. soya sauce
- ❖ 2 tbsp. ketchup
- ❖ 400-gram chicken breast
- ❖ 1 cup chopped carrot
- ❖ 1 cup peas
- ❖ 3 tbsp. sesame seeds

Directions:

Boil spaghetti as per package instruction. Drain and rinse then shift into a big bowl. Mix sesame oil, scallions, garlic, ginger, and sugar in a separate bowl. Heat over a low or medium fire until it sizzles and cook for 2 minutes. Now, turn off the flame and stir in ketchup and soy sauce. Now, add crushed and chopped carrots and shredded cheese into noodles then put it into a pan and serve!

24. Salmon tacos with pineapple salsa

Preparation time: 12 minutes | Cooking time: 15 minutes | Servings: 5

Ingredients:

- ❖ 1 pound salmon
- ❖ 1 tsp. chili powder
- ❖ ¾ tsp. salt
- ❖ 2 tbsp. olive oil
- ❖ 5 cups mixed coleslaw
- ❖ ½ lemon juice
- ❖ 6-inch corn tortillas
- ❖ ¾ cup pineapple salsa
- ❖ Chopped fresh cilantro
- ❖ Hot sauce to serve

Directions:

Place a baking sheet with foil where salmon will be below up to 3 to 4 inch. Preheat broiler until it gets completely hot. Line a baking dish with aluminum foil. Place salmon and bake one side until it gets browned and bake another afterwards to make it brown too. All fillet will take about 10 minutes to reach that point. Now sprinkle chili powder and ¼ tsp salt and place it back in the oven for 2 more minutes to let absorb inside with spices. Next, toss coleslaw onto a pan with 1 tsp. salt and 1 tbsp. olive oil. Get the salmon out and divide it among tortillas. For topping, use salsa and garnish with cilantro and serve!

25. Bake bacon French toast

*Preparation time: 15 minutes | **Cooking time:** 30 minutes | **Servings:** 5*

Ingredients:

- ❖ 8 cups cubed bread
- ❖ 8 eggs
- ❖ 2 cups of milk
- ❖ ½ tsp. cinnamon
- ❖ ½ cup packed brown sugar
- ❖ 1 pound bacon
- ❖ 1 cup shredded cheddar cheese

Directions:

Place a baking dish on slap and put bread greased with oil under butter paper. Just line up every ingredient over bread, i.e. eggs, milk brown sugar, bacon, cinnamon, and cheese. Freeze it into the refrigerator overnight. Remove it from the fridge the next day before 30 minutes to cook. Preheat oven to bake at 375F. and bake it for 1 hour until a knife goes into it and comes out clean. Hold on 10 minutes to serve as it gets to be hot.

26. Farro salad with grilled steak

Preparation time: 10 minutes | Cooking time: 10 minutes | Servings: 2

Ingredients:

- ❖ 1 can faro
- ❖ 2 medium bell peppers
- ❖ 5 tbsp. olive oil
- ❖ 500 grams of beef
- ❖ 2 cups of corn
- ❖ 1 cup kale leaves
- ❖ ¼ balsamic vinegar

Directions:

Cook farro as per instruction on the package is given. Toss bell peppers in 2 tbsp. olive oil. Grill steaks and sprinkle pepper and cook until doneness of beef. Grill the beef and stuff with all remaining crunchy peppers to taste. Toss farro with pepper. Add corn, kale leaves, balsamic vinegar, salt to taste and olive oil. Now serve with farro.

27. Chicken breast with tomato pesto

*Preparation time: 15 minutes | **Cooking Time:** 90 minutes | **Servings:** 5*

Ingredients:

- ❖ 4 chicken breasts
- ❖ ½ cup pesto sauce
- ❖ 1 cup Dijon mustard
- ❖ ¼ cup red wine vinegar
- ❖ 15 ounce roasted tomatoes
- ❖ ¼ cup chicken broth
- ❖ Salt and pepper to taste

Directions:

Let preheat oven for 15 minutes on 375 F. Grease baking dish with cooking spray and spread all chicken breast pieces. Then pour tomatoes into and season with salt and pepper, pour red wine and other remaining ingredients. Remember to place a foil underneath and cook for 80 to 85 minutes. Serve it with tomato sauce itself for a yummy and delicious meal.

28. Sheet Pan Nachos with Veggies

Preparation time: 1 hour | Cooking time: 30 - 40 minutes | Servings: 5

Ingredients:

- ❖ 1 tsp. olive oil
- ❖ 15 oz. unsalted pinto beans
- ❖ 1 clove garlic
- ❖ 4 tbsp. fresh lime juice
- ❖ 1 ½ tsp. sea salt
- ❖ 1 tsp. chili powder
- ❖ ½ tsp. ground cumin
- ❖ 16 ounce tortilla chips
- ❖ 1 cup green and red salsa
- ❖ ½ cup cilantro leaves
- ❖ 1 avocado
- ❖ 2 ounce cheddar cheese

Directions:

Have a frying pan and fry garlic in oil add all seasonings and veggies and stir fry until the color changes. Now set it aside. Separately, the toss pan get smoke to all of the seasonings. Now mix both well. Top with tortilla chips, cilantro and a ripe avocado. Spread cheese on top of everything and bake on preheated oven for 20 minutes.

29. Stir fry vegetables with teriyaki

Preparation time: 30 minutes | Cooking time: 40 minutes | Servings: 4

Ingredients:

- ❖ 2 tbsp. olive oil
- ❖ 1 medium onion
- ❖ 3 cloves crushed garlic
- ❖ 1 tbsp. ginger paste
- ❖ 2 cup carrot
- ❖ 2 bell peppers
- ❖ ¾ cup roasted salted cashews
- ❖ 1 large broccoli chopped
- ❖ 1 cup green onions
- ❖ 1 ½ cup peas
- ❖ 2 cup brown rice

For sauce:

- ❖ 1 can pineapple
- ❖ 1 cup soya sauce
- ❖ 2 tbsp. honey
- ❖ 1 tbsp. rice vinegar
- ❖ 1 tbsp. chia seeds

Directions:

For teriyaki, have oil in a toss pan on medium flame and throw onion onto it. Now add ginger garlic paste and fry well. Known mixer aroma is about to spread. Pour all veggies and cook till fry. Even pour cashews though. For sauce, first have a pineapple with juice in a pan on a low medium flame. Twist a spoon until the juice is released. Now, you need to add honey soy sauce and rice vinegar while continuously stirring with a spoon. Add seeds into the sauce. Now, pour out the sauce you need and veggies to eat. Mix in separate bowl and enjoy!

30. Quinoa Tacos

Preparation time: 20 minutes | Cooking time: 30 minutes | Servings: 5

Ingredients:

- ❖ 1 tbsp. olive oil
- ❖ 1 onion
- ❖ 2 garlic cloves
- ❖ 1 tbsp. cilantro
- ❖ 1 ½ cup Beans
- ❖ 2 cups chicken broth
- ❖ 1 tsp green chili
- ❖ 3 tomatoes
- ❖ 1 cup quinoa
- ❖ Mixed spices
- ❖ 1 cup frozen corn
- ❖ Tortillas

Directions:

Preheat oven for 10 minutes at 375F. Now grease baking dish with cooking spray and add in the quinoa. Pour all ingredients over it one at a time, including yellow onion, and the other veggies. Now in a pan on medium flame, just fry boiled beans, frozen corn. Now pour it onto fish. Season with all the spices, including the cumin, paprika and other ingredients to your preference. Bake it in the oven for 30 minutes. Top it with tortillas and serve

Chapter 7:
Recipes for Snacks & Desserts

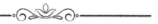

1. Blueberry cherry chip

*Preparation time: 15 minutes l **Cooking time**: 40 minutes l **Servings**: 8*

Ingredients:

- ❖ 1 cup oat meal
- ❖ 1/3 cup whole wheat flour
- ❖ ½ cup macadamia nuts
- ❖ 2 tbsp. coconut oil
- ❖ 3 tbsp. butter
- ❖ 2 tbsp. honey
- ❖ 1 tsp cinnamon
- ❖ ¼ tsp nutmeg
- ❖ 1/8 tsp salt
- ❖ 4 cup cherry frozen
- ❖ 2 cup blueberries, frozen

Directions:

First of all, preheat oven at 375 degrees, and set the baking dish by greasing with butter. Take a bowl and add oatmeal, flour, nuts and mix well. Now in a pan add coconut oil, butter, honey, cinnamon, nutmeg and salt. Stir the mixture on low flame until butter melt and mixture well combine. Cook it for 3 minutes, after that pour it on the oatmeal mixture and stir well. Set the berries and cherries in a dish and pour mixture over them with spoon. Bake them for 35 to 40 minutes or until crispy. Serve when cool down.

2. Baked apple with tahini raisin filling

*Preparation time: 15 minutes l **Cooking time:** 30 minutes l **Servings:** 4*

Ingredients:

- ❖ 4 apples
- ❖ ¾ cup tahini
- ❖ 1 cup apple juice
- ❖ 3 tbsp. raisins
- ❖ 1/3 cup pecans
- ❖ ¼ tsp cinnamon
- ❖ Nutmeg as per taste
- ❖ Vanilla as per taste
- ❖ ¾ cup water boiling

Directions:

Set the baking dish with oil grease and heat oven at 375 degrees. Cut the apples from the center to remove the core and set them in baking dish. Take a small bowl, add tahini, apple juice, cinnamon, nutmeg, and vanilla and mix them together. Now fill the center core of apples with the mixture. Pour the boiling water in baking dish, apple juice over the apples, and bake for 30 minutes. After that, remove from the oven and serve warm.

3. Pear banana nut muffins

*Preparation time: 30 minutes l **Cooking time**: 20 minutes l **Servings**: 12*

Ingredients:

- ❖ 1 pear
- ❖ 2 tbsp. pear nectar
- ❖ 1 cup whole wheat flour
- ❖ 1 cup oats
- ❖ 1 tbsp. flaxseed
- ❖ 3 tbsp. maple syrup
- ❖ 1 tsp baking powder
- ❖ ½ baking soda
- ❖ 1 tsp cinnamon
- ❖ ¼ tsp cardamom
- ❖ ¼ tsp salt
- ❖ 2 eggs
- ❖ 1/3 cup almond milk
- ❖ 2 tbsp. butter
- ❖ 2 tsp vanilla
- ❖ 1 medium banana
- ❖ 1 cup walnuts, chopped

Directions:

Preheat oven to 375F, set the muffin cup with parchment paper, and set aside. In a pan, add pear nectar and pear and boil over medium heat. When it starts to simmer, then reduce the heat and cook until smooth. Let it cool. In a bowl, add flour, oats, flaxseeds, baking soda, baking powder, cinnamon, cardamom, and salt and mix well. In another bowl, add the peach syrup, eggs, almond milk, butter, and vanilla to whisk well. Add banana and after mixing, pour it on the dry ingredients. Fold them well and pour into the muffin cups. Bake them for the 20 minutes or until well cooked and turn brown. Remove and let them cool down before serving.

4. Berry banana slush

Preparation time: 5 minutes l Cooking time: 5 minutes l Servings: 2

Ingredients:

- ❖ 2 banana
- ❖ 200 g frozen berries
- ❖ Ice cubes if required

Directions:

Take a blender and pour the mixed berries inside, including blueberries, strawberries and raspberries and blend them well until turns to a combined slush. Add ice for if you'd like to increase the slushy consistency. In serving cups, add the banana cubes, and pour the berry slush on them. Serve the chill and yummy banana berry slush.

5. Sticky toffee pudding

Preparation time: 25 minutes l Cooking time: 1 hour l Servings: 4

Ingredients:

- ❖ 175 g dates, dried
- ❖ 150 ml maple syrup
- ❖ 1 tbsp. vanilla extract
- ❖ 2 eggs
- ❖ 85g flour

Directions:

Preheat oven at 180 degrees. Take a pan add water and pour dates cook on low flame for 5 to 6 minutes. Add the dates and water into blender and pulse until turn smooth. Add maple syrup and vanilla extract and blend again. Pour the mixture into a bowl, now whisk egg into separate bowl. In dates mixture add flour, egg and fold them well until well combined. Take pudding pan and pour maple syrup into the base, now pour the mixture on it and bake for at least an hour. After that, transfer it to the serving plate, dress it with maple syrup and serve.

6. Baked apple with cinnamon & ginger

*Preparation time: 10 minutes l **Cooking time:** 40 minutes l **Servings:** 4*

Ingredients:

- ❖ 4 apples
- ❖ 2 ginger, chopped
- ❖ ½ tsp cinnamon
- ❖ 4 prunes, chopped
- ❖ 50 g muscovado sugar
- ❖ 1 tbsp. butter
- ❖ 4 scoops vanilla ice cream for serving

Directions:

Preheat oven to 200F. Cut the quarter of each apple and set them into a baking dish. Take a bowl, add ginger, cinnamon, sugar, prunes and butter, and mix well. Pour the mixture over the apples and put the butter on each apple top. Bake them for 35 minutes or until cooked well. Remove and serve the hot baked cinnamon apple with a scoop of vanilla ice cream.

7. Chocolate muffin with chocolate custard

*Preparation time: 10 minutes l **Cooking time:** 10 minutes l **Servings:** 6*

Ingredients:

- ❖ 1 tbsp. cocoa powder
- ❖ 100 g raising flour
- ❖ ½ tsp baking soda
- ❖ 50 g caster sugar
- ❖ 100 ml skimmed milk
- ❖ 1 egg
- ❖ 2 tbsp. sunflower oil
- ❖ 150g low fat custard
- ❖ 25g dark chocolate

Directions:

Preheat the oven and set the muffin tray by greasing it with oil. In a large bowl, add flour, cocoa powder, sugar, soda, and mix well. In another bowl, whisk eggs, milk, oil and mix together. Pour the mixture on dry ingredients and make a fine batter. Now, pour the mixture with the help of a spoon on the muffins tray and bake for 10 to 15 minutes or until cooked and turned brown. While they are in the oven, pour custard into a pan and add dark chocolate into it or stir until combined and smooth. When the muffins are done, put it onto the serving plate, pour hot custard over it, and serve hot.

8. Lighter Apple & pear pie

Preparation time: 20 minutes *l* **Cooking time:** 40 minutes *l* **Servings:** 6

Ingredients:

- ❖ 6 apples
- ❖ 4 pears
- ❖ 1 lemon juice & zest
- ❖ 3 tbsp. syrup
- ❖ 1 tsp mix spice
- ❖ 1 tbsp. corn flour
- ❖ 4 pastry sheets
- ❖ 4 tsp rapeseed oil
- ❖ 25g almond

Directions:

Take a pan, add apples and pears with water, syrup, lemon and mixed spices, and cook for 5 minutes. Now, remove the fruit and pour it into a pie dish and cook the remainder for another 5 minutes. Mash the remaining fruits into a mixture until smooth and until the syrup is thick in consistency. Cook that syrup for another 4 to 5 minutes and then pour it into a pie dish. Set the pastry sheets in the dish and brush oil on the top. Bake it for 30 minutes in a preheated oven at 180 degrees, until it turns brown and is cooked. Serve immediately!

9. Peach & blueberry yogurt cake

*Preparation time: 20 minutes l **Cooking time:** 1 hour l*
Servings: 10

Ingredients:

- ❖ 1 ½ cup all-purpose flour
- ❖ 1 tsp baking powder
- ❖ ½ tsp baking soda
- ❖ 2 oz. butter
- ❖ 1 cup sugar
- ❖ 2 eggs
- ❖ ½ tsp vanilla
- ❖ ½ cup yogurt
- ❖ 2 peaches, sliced
- ❖ 6 oz. blueberries
- ❖ 1 tsp sugar

Directions:

Grease the baking pan with parchment paper and set aside, preheat the oven to 350 degrees. Take a bowl, add flour, baking powder and soda. In a separate bowl, whisk eggs, butter, and sugar until fluffy. Now add vanilla extract and Greek yogurt and continue beating until well combined and the texture becomes smooth. Pour the mixture into a flour bowl and mix until well combined. Pour the batter into baking pan, set the slices of peach and sprinkle blueberries with sugar. Bake it for 30 to 35 minutes or until golden brown. When baking is done, let it cool down for 30 minutes and then serve with the yogurt topping.

10. Dark chocolate cheese bar

*Preparation time: 15 minutes l **Cooking time:** 1 hour l Servings: 12*

Ingredients:

- ❖ 1 cup cracker crumbs
- ❖ ¼ cup coconut flour
- ❖ ¼ cup cocoa powder
- ❖ 8 tbsp. cream cheese
- ❖ 2 tbsp. honey
- ❖ 1 tsp vanilla extract
- ❖ 2 to 3 tbsp. almond milk
- ❖ 1/3 cup dark chocolate chips
- ❖ 1 tsp coconut oil

Directions:

Set up a tray with the parchment paper and set it aside. Take a bowl and add graham cracker crumbs, coconut flour, and cocoa powder, and add them into a mixture. Then pour honey, vanilla extract and cream cheese. Mix them well to turn then into a fine dough. Gradually add the almond milk to make the dough soft and do not let it dry. When it's done, set it into a baking pan with the help of spatula. In a small bowl, add chocolate chips and coconut oil and set it into the microwave until melted and smooth. Pour the chocolate over the batter and set it evenly. Now put the tray into the fridge for some time until the ingredients set well. Now serve the fine dark chocolate cheese bar.

11. Skinny chocolate chip cheesecake bar

*Preparation time: 15 minutes l **Cooking time:** 35 minutes l **Servings:** 16*

Ingredients:

- ❖ ¾ cup graham cracker crumbs.
- ❖ 2 tbsp. butter
- ❖ 8 oz. cream cheese
- ❖ ¾ cup Greek yogurt
- ❖ 2 eggs
- ❖ ¼ cup sugar
- ❖ 2 tbsp. flour
- ❖ 1 tbsp. lemon juice
- ❖ 2 tbsp. vanilla extract
- ❖ ½ cup chocolate chips

Directions:

Preheat the oven to 350F and set the baking tray by setting parchment paper and set aside. In a blender, add cracker crumbs and pour butter to blend well. Transfer the mixture into a baking tray and set it with a spatula and bake for 8 to 10 minutes. In a mixer, add cream cheese and beat for a minute. Now add yogurt, egg, sugar, and flour and mix until smooth. Add the lemon juice and mix well. Now pour the mixture into a bowl and add chocolate chips and fold them well. Cover the baked crust with the cream cheese filling and bake for 20 to 25 minutes until cooked. After that, let it cool down and serve hot or chilled.

12. Frozen fruit skewers

Preparation time: 30 minutes l Cooking time: 0 l Servings: 12

Ingredients:

- ❖ ¼ of watermelon, cubed
- ❖ ½ cantaloupe, cubed
- ❖ ½ pineapple, cubed
- ❖ 1 cup grapes
- ❖ 6 oz. blueberries
- ❖ 2 to 3 banana, sliced
- ❖ 4 oz. chocolate chips

Directions:

Take the fruits and cut them in evenly into cubes. Thread the fruit alternatively on the skewers. Now cover the skewers with a plastic sheet and put in them in the refrigerator until ready to serve. In a bowl, add chocolate chips and melt in a microwave for 2 to 3 minutes until smooth. Let the chocolate cool down a bit. Remove the fruit skewers and drizzle the melted chocolate over the fruit skewers. Now put it into refrigerator and let it freeze. Serve frozen fruit skewer immediately!

13. Whole wheat chocolate cake donuts

Preparation time: 5 minutes l Cooking time: 15 minutes l Servings: 6

Ingredients:

- ❖ ¾ cup almond milk
- ❖ 1 tsp lemon juice
- ❖ 1 cup whole wheat flour
- ❖ 2 tbsp. sugar
- ❖ 2 tsp cocoa powder
- ❖ ½ tsp baking powder
- ❖ ½ tsp baking soda
- ❖ ½ tsp salt
- ❖ ½ tbsp. flax seed
- ❖ 2 tbsp. oil
- ❖ 1 cup sugar, powdered
- ❖ 1 tsp vanilla extract
- ❖ 1 tbsp. milk

Directions:

Preheat oven at 350F and set the donut baking tray. In a small bowl, mix the almond milk with lemon juice and set aside for 5 minutes. In a bowl, add flour, flaxseed, sugar, cocoa powder, baking powder, baking soda, salt, oil ,and mix them well. Now pour the almond milk and lemon mixture into it and mix it until combined. Pour the batter over the donut baking tray and bake for 10 to 13 minutes or until fluffy and cooked. Remove them and let them cool down. Sprinkle powdered sugar or milk. Serve immediately or store for later use.

14. Blueberry and cream dessert

*Preparation time: 30 minutes l **Cooking time:** 15 minutes l **Servings:***

Ingredients:

- ❖ 12 oz. blueberries, frozen
- ❖ 2 tbsp. sugar
- ❖ 2 tbsp. cornstarch
- ❖ ¼ cup water
- ❖ 1 tbsp. lemon juice
- ❖ 16 oz. light cream cheese
- ❖ 2/3 cup dried milk
- ❖ 2/3 cup granulated sugar
- ❖ 1 ½ heavy cream
- ❖ 3 tbsp. powdered sugar

Directions:

Take a pan and add water, blueberries, sugar, cornstarch and lemon juice. Bring it to a boil and simmer for 5 to 7 minutes over a medium flame. Let it cool down to room temperature. For the cake and cream layer, take a blender, add cream cheese, milk, sugar and blend until smooth and creamy. Fold the cream cheese mixture with the cake cubes until well combined. Mix the heavy cream with sugar for the whipped cream until it turns soft and fluffy. In a serving cup, fill it with the mixture, and add blueberry syrup and another layer of cream cheese cake. After that, dress it with the whipped cream and put it in the refrigerator for 2 hours to set and chill it. Serve the chilled blueberry cream dessert.

15. Cream cheese lemon coffee cake

Preparation time: 20 *minutes* l *Cooking time:* 40 *minutes* l *Servings:* 16

Ingredients:

- ❖ 8 oz. cream cheese
- ❖ ¼ cup sugar
- ❖ 2 egg
- ❖ 2 tsp lemon juice
- ❖ 1 ½ cup flour
- ❖ ½ tsp baking powder
- ❖ ¼ tsp baking soda
- ❖ ¼ tsp salt
- ❖ ½ cup vegetable oil
- ❖ ¾ cup granulated sugar
- ❖ ½ cup Greek yogurt
- ❖ 1 lemon zest
- ❖ Powdered sugar for dust

Directions:

Preheat oven to 350F and set the parchment paper in a baking try and grease it with oil. In a bowl, add cream cheese, sugar, egg and lemon juice, mix the ingredients until well combined and turn smooth. In another bowl, add flour, baking powder, baking soda and salt and mix them together. In blender, add egg, oil and sugar and blend until smooth. Add yogurt, lemon zest and lemon juice and make a fine mixture. After that, add the flour gradually into the mixture and continue mixing on a medium speed. When the mixture is well combined, pour it into a baking tray and set well. Pour the cream cheese mixture over it and set well. Bake it for 40 to 45 minutes or until cooked. Remove it from the oven and let it cool down. Cut into slices and serve.

16. Baked pears with walnuts and honey

*Preparation time: 5 minutes l **Cooking time:** 25 minutes l **Servings:** 4*

Ingredients:

- ❖ 2 pears
- ❖ ¼ cup honey
- ❖ ¼ tsp cinnamon
- ❖ ¼ tsp vanilla extract
- ❖ Salt as per taste
- ❖ ¼ cup walnuts

Directions:

First of all, preheat the oven to 400F and set the parchment paper into the baking tray and set aside. Slice the pear from the center with a knife and remove the seeds. Set the pears into a baking tray over parchment paper. In a bowl, add cinnamon, honey, salt and vanilla extract and mix well. With a spoon, pour the mixture over the pears evenly and bake for the 20 to 25 minutes. Remove when cooked well, then garnish with walnuts and honey over the pears and serve.

17. Apple baked chips

Preparation time: 5 minute' l Cooking time: 1 hour, 20 minutes l Servings: 1 bowl

Ingredients:

- ❖ 3 large apples
- ❖ 1 tsp cinnamon
- ❖ 2 tsp sugar
- ❖ 1 tsp olive oil

Directions:

First of all, preheat the oven to 200F and set the baking tray with parchment paper and set it aside. With a sharp knife, cut the apple to remove its core from center and make round slices. Set the apple slices on parchment paper, spray olive oil, and apply cinnamon and sugar to each slice. Bake the apples for 40 minutes. Now remove and flip the side and add some cinnamon or cook again for 40 minutes. Let them become golden brown and crispy. Remove and let them cool. These can be stored for 3 days.

18. Banana, honey & peanut butter roll

Preparation time: l Cooking time: l Servings:

Ingredients:

- ❖ 1 flatbread
- ❖ 1 tbsp. peanut butter
- ❖ ½ banana
- ❖ ½ tbsp. honey

Directions:

Take banana and cut into slices. On a flatbread, spread the peanut butter with the help of knife and spread evenly. Place the banana chunks on top and pour some honey over top. Make a roll of the bread and cut the center in half. Serve with milk or enjoy plain for a snack.

19. Blueberry oatmeal Greek yogurt muffins

*Preparation time: 10 minutes l **Cooking time**: 30 minutes l **Servings**: 6*

Ingredients:

- ❖ 1 cup all-purpose flour
- ❖ 1 cup oats
- ❖ 2 tsp baking powder
- ❖ ¼ tsp salt
- ❖ 2 eggs
- ❖ 1 cup plain yogurt
- ❖ 1/3 cup honey
- ❖ ¼ cup milk
- ❖ 2 tsp vanilla extract
- ❖ 1 cup blueberries

Directions:

Preheat the oven to 350F and set the parchment paper into a muffin tray and set aside. Separate 1tbsp flour aside. In a bowl, add the rest of the flour, oats, baking powder and salt. In another bowl, whisk the eggs, yogurt, honey, milk and vanilla extract. After that, pour the flour into the mixture and fold them well until combined. Add blueberries into it and mix well. Pour the mixture into muffin cups evenly. Bake for 20 minutes or until golden and cooked. Take them out and let them cool. Sprinkle some flour or serve with a yogurt topping.

20. Caprese salad

Preparation time: 5 minutes l Cooking time: 5 minutes l Servings: 1

Ingredients:

- ❖ 1 tbsp. balsamic vinegar
- ❖ 1 tomato
- ❖ ½ tbsp. olive oil
- ❖ 1 oz. mozzarella
- ❖ 1 ½ leaves of basil
- ❖ Salt & pepper to taste

Directions:

Take the tomato, and wash and cut it into slices. In a medium bowl, add the tomato, vinegar, olive oil, salt and pepper and toss them well until combined. Now add mozzarella and mix well. Sprinkle some basil leaves on top and serve.

21. Chickpeas with white toast

*Preparation time: 5 minutes l **Cooking time:** 5 minutes l Servings: 1*

Ingredients:

- ❖ 1 slice of white bread
- ❖ ¼ cup chickpeas, boiled
- ❖ 3 tbsp. grated carrot
- ❖ 1 tsp olive oil
- ❖ 1 lemon juice
- ❖ Salt & pepper to taste

Directions:

Take a small bowl and add chickpeas and mash them with the help of a fork. Now, add olive oil, lemon juice, carrot chunks and salt or pepper to your taste. Mix them well until combined. Take a slice of toast and apply the mixture on the toast with a knife. Sprinkle some carrot on top and serve as a healthy snack.

22. Baked zucchini chips

*Preparation time: 10 minutes l **Cooking time:** 2 hours l **Servings:** 1 bowl*

Ingredients:

- ❖ 1 zucchini
- ❖ 2 tbsp. olive oil
- ❖ Salt to taste

Directions:

To begin, preheat the oven to 225F and set the parchment paper in a baking tray and set it aside. Take zucchini and cut it into round slices with 2 to 3 of thickness. Set the zucchini slices on the baking tray and cover it with a paper towel, set another layer and again cover it with a towel. It helps to absorb the extra moisture while baking. Press the zucchini slice well between a towel so the moisture will absorb. Now brush the olive oil on each slice and sprinkle some salt. Bake them in a preheated oven for 2 hours or until they turn brown or turn crispy. Serve when they cool down or store for up to 2 days.

23. White bean salad

*Preparation time: 5 minutes l **Cooking time:** 5 minutes l Servings: 2*

Ingredients:

- ❖ 1 cup white beans
- ❖ ½ cucumber
- ❖ 1 tomato
- ❖ Handful of dill
- ❖ ½ lemon juice
- ❖ 1 cup white beans
- ❖ ¼ cup vinegar
- ❖ Salt as per taste

Directions:

In a pan full of water, boil the white beans until soft and cooked. Now, drain out the water and set them aside. Wash the tomato and cucumber and cut it into cubes. Take a medium bowl and add cucumber, tomato, dill, lemon juice, vinegar and boiled white beans. Now mix them well. Sprinkle some salt as per your taste and toss to combine. Serve the refreshing white bean salad as a snack.

24. Banana pudding cookie

Preparation time: 5 *minutes* l *Cooking time:* 10 *minutes* l *Servings:* 12

Ingredients:

- ❖ 3 bananas
- ❖ 1 egg
- ❖ 3 tablespoons unsalted butter
- ❖ 2/3 cup plain flour
- ❖ 1 teaspoon vanilla
- ❖ 3 tablespoons plain yogurt
- ❖ 1 teaspoon baking powder
- ❖ ¼ cup Sugar
- ❖ ¼ teaspoon salt
- ❖ 1 pack vanilla pudding mix

Directions:

In a bowl, add mashed bananas and baking soda. Mix it well and set aside. Beat egg, and add cream, sugar, yogurt, and butter in it and whisk it. In another bowl, mix pudding mix, flour, and salt and add this mixture to the cream mixture and whisk well. In the end, add the banana mixture in it and combine well. Now, on the greased baking dish, scoop the batter in the form of cookies. Bake in for 10 minutes in the preheated oven on the temperature of 350F.

25. Vanilla cupcake

*Preparation time: 10 minutes l **Cooking time**: 20 minutes l **Servings**: 12*

Ingredients:

- ❖ 2 cups flour¾ cup sugar
- ❖ 2 eggs
- ❖ 1 teaspoon vanilla extract
- ❖ 1 teaspoon baking soda
- ❖ 1 cup milk
- ❖ ½ cup butter
- ❖ ½ teaspoon salt

Directions:

Preheat the oven to 375F. Prepare the muffin tins with a liner. In a bowl, whisk butter and sugar and add eggs one by one. Add all the remaining items and mix well. Pour the batter in the muffin tins and bake it in the preheated oven for around 18 minutes and serve it.

26. White chocolate and strawberry tart

*Preparation time: 15 minutes l **Cooking time**: 10 minutes l **Servings**: 2*

Ingredients:

- ❖ 5 teaspoon melted butter
- ❖ 1 cup ground shortbread cookies
- ❖ 3 tablespoons cream
- ❖ ¾ cup fresh sliced strawberries
- ❖ 1 1/3 cups melted butter
- ❖ 1 ½ cups grated white chocolate
- ❖ 2 tablespoons chocolate chips

Directions:

Prepare a baking tray with a greased baking liner. Mix the crumble cookers and butter and pour it in the baking dish and press it properly from every side. Bake it for 10 minutes at a 350F temperature. Microwave the beaten cream for 20 seconds and add white chocolate in it and whisk. Pour this filling on the baked crust and add chocolate chips and strawberries on its top.

27. Baileys custard

Preparation time: 2 minutes l Cooking time: 10 minutes l Servings: 4

Ingredients:

- ❖ 4 egg yolks
- ❖ 3 ½ cups cream
- ❖ ½ cup baileys can
- ❖ ¼ cup sugar
- ❖ 1 teaspoon vanilla extract
- ❖ ½ cup milk

Directions:

Take a bowl and mix all the ingredients thoroughly. Now put it in a pot and cook over 90C temperature for approximately 10 minutes. You can serve it immediately or can serve it cold. For cooling it keep it in the refrigerator for some time and present it.

28. Mexican bean salad

Preparation time: 15 minutes l **Chilling time:** 1-hour l
Servings: 8

Ingredients:

- ❖ 15 ounce rinsed and drained black beans
- ❖ 1 chopped green bell pepper
- ❖ 1 chopped onion
- ❖ 1 chopped red bell pepper
- ❖ 15 ounce rinsed and drained kidney beans
- ❖ ½ cup olive oil
- ❖ 10 ounce cooked corn
- ❖ 2 tablespoons lemon juice
- ❖ 2 chicken breasts
- ❖ ½ cup vinegar
- ❖ 1 minced garlic
- ❖ 2 tablespoons sugar
- ❖ ½ tablespoon ground black pepper
- ❖ ½ tablespoon ground cumin
- ❖ 15 ounce rinsed and drained cannellini beans

Directions:

Take a bowl and add all the wet ingredients. Mix them well and add the remaining ingredients in it. Whisk all the ingredients until they combine well. Put it in the refrigerator for an hour and serve.

29. Peanut butter no bake cookies

*Preparation time: 10 minutes l **Cooking time**: 1 hour l Servings: 14 cookies*

Ingredients:

- ❖ ½ cup peanut butter
- ❖ 1 banana
- ❖ 1/3 cup maple syrup
- ❖ 1 ½ cup quinoa flakes
- ❖ ¼ cup milk
- ❖ 1/8 tsp salt
- ❖ ½ cup dark chocolate

Directions:

Set the parchment paper into a baking tray and set it aside. In a bowl, add peanut butter and banana and mash well. Take a pan and add maple syrup or peanut butter and banana mixture to cook for 2 minutes until combined. Take off the flame and add quinoa flakes, milk, and salt and mix. Let the mixture cool down for about 10 minutes. Meanwhile, melt the dark chocolate in a microwave and fold it into the mixture. Use a scope and make round balls and then flatten them into the shape of cookies. Place the cookies over the parchment paper and leave them into refrigerator for 1 hour. Serve when set and chilled.

30. Cucumber roll ups

*Preparation time: 5 minutes l **Cooking time**: 10 minutes l **Servings**: 12*

Ingredients:

- ❖ 1 lb. tomatoes
- ❖ 1 cucumber
- ❖ ½ onion
- ❖ 2 avocados
- ❖ 2 tbsp. olive oil
- ❖ 2 tbsp. vinegar
- ❖ 1 tbsp. honey
- ❖ ½ tsp salt
- ❖ ¼ tsp black pepper

Directions:

Wash the tomatoes and cucumber and cut them with a knife. Slice the cucumber into long slices. Similarly, cut and mash the avocados. Take a bowl add the avocado mixture, tomatoes, olive oil, honey, salt, pepper, and vinegar. Mix them all together well and set aside. Take the cucumber slices and apply the mixture over them and then roll up the slices. Serve the cucumber roll ups as a snack and enjoy.

Conclusion

Acid reflux is a stomach related or digestive disorder that creates irritation and a restless condition for a person. The main reason behind this issue is poor digestion, improper food intake, lack of sleep, and inactivity. An increase in obesity and other health complications can cause acid reflux. In this chronic disorder, a person feels heartburn and feels like their food is not properly being digested. Stomach acid and food reverse into the food canal that causes an inability to perform the task and continuous burp can affect a person's productivity as well.

As per the consultants, it is necessary to treat the acid reflux at the initial stage with food intake, exercise, and diet control by reducing the weight or following proper medication. It not treated well, then it may cause further health complications like cancer or ulcers as well. To get quick relief from acid reflux, it is necessary to adopt certain dietary changes like taking small meals instead of full meals, following an exercise routine, reducing citrus intake, limiting spicy and fried food intake, and reducing weight. At the initial stage of acid reflux, it can be treated and prevented with healthy and organic food choices. It also requires a proper medical checkup; this helps to find out how severe the problem is. Consulting doctors and taking their advice for the treatment and precautions is a necessary step a person has to take to avoid gastric acid reflux. In this book, a number of healthy and organic recipes are mentioned that will help a person to enjoy good food and relief in acid reflux conditions as well.

Made in the USA
Middletown, DE
07 December 2020